Wandering the Wards

Wandering the Wards provides a detailed and unflinching ethnographic examination of life within the contemporary hospital. It reveals the institutional and ward cultures that inform the organisation and delivery of everyday care for one of the largest populations within them: people living with dementia who require urgent unscheduled hospital care.

Drawing on five years of research embedded in acute wards in the UK, the authors follow people living with dementia through their admission, shadowing hospital staff as they interact with them during and across shifts. In a major contribution to the tradition of hospital ethnography, this book provides a valuable analysis of the organisation and delivery of routine care and everyday interactions at the bedside, which reveal the powerful continuities and durability of ward cultures of care and their impacts on people living with dementia.

Katie Featherstone is a Reader in Sociology and Medicine at the School of Healthcare Sciences at Cardiff University, UK.

Andy Northcott is a Senior Lecturer at the Leicester School of Allied Health Sciences at De Montfort University, UK.

Routledge Studies in Health and Medical Anthropology

Depression in Kerala
Ayurveda and Mental Health Care in 21st-Century India
Claudia Lang

Diagnosis Narratives and the Healing Ritual in Western Medicine
James P. Meza

Haemophilia in Aotearoa New Zealand
Julie Park, Kathryn M. Scott, Deon York, and Michael Carnahan

The Anthropology of Epidemics
Christos Lynteris, Frédéric Keck and Ann H. Kelly

Locating Zika
Social Change and Governance in an Age of Mosquito Pandemics
Edited by Kevin Bardosh

Affective Health and Masculinities in South Africa
An Ethnography of (In)vulnerability
Hans Reihling

Wandering the Wards
An Ethnography of Hospital Care and its Consequences for People Living with Dementia
Katie Featherstone and Andy Northcott

www.routledge.com/Routledge-Studies-in-Health-and-Medical-Anthropology/book-series/RSHMA

Wandering the Wards

An Ethnography of Hospital Care and its Consequences for People Living with Dementia

Katie Featherstone and Andy Northcott

Routledge
Taylor & Francis Group
LONDON AND NEW YORK

First published 2021
by Routledge
2 Park Square, Milton Park, Abingdon, Oxon OX14 4RN

and by Routledge
52 Vanderbilt Avenue, New York, NY 10017

Routledge is an imprint of the Taylor & Francis Group, an informa business

British Library Cataloguing-in-Publication Data
A catalogue record for this book is available from the British Library

Library of Congress Cataloging-in-Publication Data
Names: Featherstone, Katie, author. | Northcott, Andy, author.
Title: Wandering the wards : an ethnography of hospital care and its consequences for people living with dementia / Katie Featherstone and Andy Northcott.
Description: New York : Routledge, 2020. | Series: Routledge studies in health and medical anthropology | Includes bibliographical references and index.
Identifiers: LCCN 2020029499 (print) | LCCN 2020029500 (ebook) |
Subjects: LCSH: Dementia--Patients--Care. | Dementia--Patients--Care--Great Britain.
Classification: LCC RC521 .F43 2020 (print) | LCC RC521 (ebook) | DDC 616.8/31--dc23
LC record available at https://lccn.loc.gov/2020029499
LC ebook record available at https://lccn.loc.gov/2020029500

ISBN: 978-1-350-07845-1 (hbk)
ISBN: 978-1-003-08733-5 (ebk)

Typeset in Times New Roman
by SPi Global, India

To Nick, Jerry, and Louie

Contents

Preface

This book is the culmination of the five years we have spent wandering these wards, exploring the everyday organisation and delivery of work within them, to examine the experiences and consequences for the significant population of people living with dementia admitted within them. Our research could not have happened without the support of the hospital staff, the nurses, healthcare assistants, auxiliary and administrative staff, therapists and medical teams who were so warm, open and receptive in welcoming two strangers into their workplace to observe, shadow, and essentially to follow them around with a note pad and pen. Nor would it have been possible without the many people living with dementia, their families and friends who were willing to let us observe their care, to join them at the bedside, to speak to us and share their deeply personal stories and experiences.

Our research is publicly funded and has been supported by grants from the National Institute of Health Research Health Services and Delivery Research (NIHR HS&DR) funding programme. They have funded Katie as Principal Investigator, and Andy as co-applicant and researcher across two projects since 2015, and continue to fund and support our research. The work presented in this book is drawn largely from our experiences during our first ethnography, exploring 'The management of refusal of food, drink and medications by people with dementia admitted to hospital with an acute condition' (NIHR HS&DR project number 13/10/80) but also draws on elements of our second ethnography 'Understanding how to facilitate continence for people living with dementia in acute hospital settings: raising awareness and improving care' (NIHR HS&DR project number 15/136/67). We were wandering the wards for this second study during the writing of this book and this enabled us to deepen, test, and refine our analysis. This funding has given us the opportunity to spend 330 days within wards in 8 hospitals across England and Wales, almost a full calendar year, exploring and understanding the social processes and the cultures of care that inform the organisation and delivery of everyday bedside care that we present in this book.

The start of our involvement

Our own awareness of the impacts and experiences of people living with dementia within our wards happened by chance. We were invited to join a research development meeting with clinicians from the medical and surgical teams within a large regional teaching hospital to discuss what they described as the 'problem' of dementia in their wards. The room was full and there was an animated debate about the best solution; the focus was on finding a potential 'off the shelf' intervention they could use and evaluate in their acute wards. We repeated a number of times: could they tell us what the key problem was? In the midst of intense debate, no one seemed to be listening and so tuning out we turned to our neighbour, who was the only dementia specialist nurse within this 1000-bed hospital. We still didn't understand the issue and as we talked it became clear to her that we assumed she worked within one 30-bed specialist ward caring for people living with dementia, who had been admitted because they required specialist support and could no longer be cared for in the community. She viewed us with a mixture of exasperation, frustration, and weariness, and explained that no, almost 50% of the patients across the acute wards in this hospital were also living with dementia. This was the pivot point where the focus for our research programme became clear.

Involving carers and people living with dementia

At this very early development stage we relied on carers, who confirmed that the acute setting was an important site where research was needed, and where care quality was a pressing issue having a significant impact on their partners living with dementia. We were introduced to a local group of carers who kindly invited us to meet up with them. Over lots of tea and cake one afternoon, we asked them if hospital care was an issue for them. From our notes at the time, they all described the hospital as 'the worst experience', 'scary', 'horrendous', and 'a very bad time'. Key factors for them included feelings of staff not listening to them, not respecting their experience or expertise in looking after their partner who was living with dementia and not considering their specific needs. They believed their partner was typically in worse health, with their condition significantly deteriorating following an admission. They reported having lots of work to do to help their partners recover from a stay on an acute ward, regaining skills and independence (particularly the loss of mobility and walking, continence, and sleeping patterns) that had been lost during their admission. They reported that in their experience, people living with dementia were expected to conform and to behave 'normally' within wards. They described to us how failure to conform often resulted in further sanctions, including security guards being called and stationed at a person's bedside. This was the start of a longer-term collaboration with this group and a large network of carers, which have become more enduring friendships.

Throughout our ethnography, at every stage we have involved carers and people living with dementia in the priority setting, development, planning, analysis, and governance of our research. They have also been closely involved in our ongoing efforts to use these findings to develop and test interventions to support acute wards and improve care. We have involved them formally as co-applicants in our funding applications, and as part of our research governance through membership of our research management group, carers' steering group, and external oversight committee.

Throughout this time, we have also carried out a series of public consultation events with people living with dementia and family carers, which is ongoing. During these events, we discovered that our findings strongly resonated. This work represents a form of member checking or respondent validation and their recognition of the ward cultures we present and examine, support the reliability and validity of our fieldwork and analysis.

Systematic inequalities

When we began exploring what was already known about hospital care we were immediately struck by the significant number of government reports, audits, and enquiries published over the last decade that together establish a consistent experience. This patient population receive poor care in hospital, to the extent that currently every person living with dementia (in England) will receive poor care at some point during their hospital admission (Care Quality Commission 2014). Importantly, this provided insights into these cultures of care and tells us that there is something deeply systematic about the inequalities people living with dementia experience, as we will explore within this book.

This growing body of work also suggests that these inequalities are an intractable issue. The poor outcomes and experiences of this population are continually being reported, yet the systems that produce them seem incredibly resistant to change. We see this as deeply connected to the invisibility of both people living with dementia and of frontline staff within acute hospital wards. There is a clear disconnect that exists between the policy directives that recognise the need for change, innovation, and improvement, and the enduring stasis and durability of these ward cultures. It is surprising that, despite the continuous transformations observable more widely within biomedicine, and the many interventions, techniques, and technologies, entering the contemporary hospital, there has been little impact on improving the organisation and delivery of timetabled care at the bedside.

In the context of the increasing demands on hospital services and their changing in-patient population, the acute setting and the field of nursing has typically reacted to reports and recommendations of the need for improving care quality, with a recognition of the need for change and innovation. Despite this, there are still widespread failures in recognising and supporting frontline staff. One of our goals was to provide a detailed understanding of ward cultures and its consequences that could provide the evidence base to inform such improvements and to ensure they support both patients and staff.

During every ward rotation we observed staff, often working in poor conditions, where understaffing was expected. Here they talked of being in a 'war zone', of physical and emotional exhaustion and burnout, of coming close to fainting from the heat and the pace of work, of crying in the sluice rooms. At the same time, staff would often go the extra mile for their patients, taking shorter breaks or staying after the end of their shift to support colleagues with a patient that needed urgent care. However, organisational cultures seemed disconnected from this and appeared unwilling or unable to recognise or value this work. We feel that the origins of this disconnect can be traced back to the earlier periods of the modern hospital.

Our ethnographic approach

This context informed our ethnographic focus on examining cultures of care within acute wards. Hospitals, particularly Euro-American hospitals and wards, appear to have received relatively little attention from contemporary ethnographers (van der Geest and Finkler 2004, Long et al. 2008). For our inspiration, we looked further back, to the pioneering institutional ethnographies that focussed on the hospital and the work of the ward: to Julius Roth (1963), Roth and Elizabeth Eddy (1967), Rose Laub Coser (1962), Alfred Stanton and Morris Schwartz (1954), Isabel Menzies Lyth ([1959] 1988), and, to a lesser extent, Willian Caudill (1958), Renee Fox (1959) and Eviater Zerubavel (1979). We understand that no hospital is the same as another, nor any ward in a given hospital quite the same as its neighbour. Yet while there was significant variation across time, specialism, location, and population, we felt a recognition of and connection to our experiences and analysis of ward life powerfully within all of these ethnographies that transcended geographical place and time period.

Involving these wards and sites

Throughout this monograph we will often refer to 'these wards'; in doing so, we are referencing an amalgamation of the cultures and practices viewed within and across these eight hospitals in England and Wales. Within this book we focus on our first period of fieldwork, exploring ten wards in the first five hospitals that allowed us to observe the everyday work within them. We also partially draw on the second phase of fieldwork carried out in six wards within three further hospitals during the writing of the book. Given that one of our goals was to provide a detailed understanding of care and its consequences that could provide the evidence base to inform improvements, we felt a strategy of examining care across a range of institutions would enhance the potential for our findings to be recognised as credible and valid by public policy, hospital institutions, and frontline staff.

Our ethnographic fieldwork and analysis were informed by the analytic tradition of grounded theory (Glaser and Strauss 1967), which supported our focus on examining the phenomena of 'dementia' and the care of people living with dementia, rather than a broad and unfocussed description of the setting itself (Charmaz 2014). The aim of our approach was to uncover the relevant conditions of people with dementia within the acute hospital setting and to understand how both they and the wide range of social actors within these settings (nurses, healthcare assistants, and the large number of hospital staff and specialisms they will come into contact with during their admission) actively shape the social world of these wards. Ethnography allows us to examine these elements, but also, importantly, the interplay between them. Our emphasis was on the organisational features of these wards and the interactional work of everyday bedside care, with the aim to access the unspoken and tacitly understood, and importantly paying attention to communication that is embodied, which may be particularly important in understanding the experiences of people living with dementia within these wards (Kontos 2012).

We utilised the constant comparative method whereby fieldwork, theoretical sampling, and analysis were interrelated (Glaser and Strauss 1967, Corbin and Strauss 1990) and carried out concurrently (Green 1998, Suddaby 2006). Preliminary analysis of fieldwork within individual sites informed the focus of later stages of sampling, fieldwork, and analysis. The flexible nature of this approach was important, because we felt it allowed us to increase the 'analytic incisiveness' (Charmaz and Mitchell 2001:160) of our ethnography.

These hospitals were purposefully selected through theoretical sampling to represent a range of hospitals types, geographies (each served a wider region covering both urban and rural populations), socio-economic catchment areas, and the interventions put into place by institutions at an organisational level to support the care of people living with dementia. We also wanted to capture the 'average' and the everyday, and each hospital in our study was selected in part because they were unremarkable. We were careful to select institutions that had not been identified by the independent regulator as failing or in special measures[1].

Within each of the first five hospitals, we focused on two types of acute wards that can be found within every hospital and known to admit large numbers of people living with dementia: five trauma and orthopaedic wards, and five medical assessment units. Trauma and orthopaedic wards are where patients are transferred, typically from an admission via accident and emergency (A&E), with a fracture. The largest contingent of patients within these wards are older people who have in layman's term broken their hip, usually following what was always described as 'a fall', or in medical terms, had sustained a neck of femur fracture. These wards were sometimes referred to as 'the NoF ward' due to this overwhelmingly being the cause of admission. While a common acute admitting condition for older people and people living with dementia, these types of fractures typically require surgical intervention, a significant period of admission within the ward, including considerable time for post-operative rehabilitation.

Assessment units go by a variety of names, but most commonly are given the title of the Medical Assessment Unit, or 'MAU'. These units are a key site for unscheduled admissions within these hospitals. The patient caseload within MAU represents a range of demographics and admitting conditions and it is where people with medical conditions are admitted by referral from their GP, from long-term community care settings, or following triage from the emergency department. Patients are admitted to these units for the assessment and stabilisation of their medical conditions and are then discharged or transferred within the hospital to a specialist acute service. Unlike trauma and orthopaedic wards, where admissions can be measured in weeks and sometimes (although less common) months, an admission to MAU typically lasts anywhere from between 12 to 48 hours, although we observed far longer admissions for people living with dementia within this setting (in some cases lasting up to 10 days). This service model is intended to facilitate patient 'flow' and improve the speed of patient assessment, and their subsequent transfer or discharge. They are typically very noisy, with more equipment and machinery and a large number of staff. As well as the staff based within the unit, there are large numbers of medical teams and specialisms from across the hospital entering this setting to assess specific patients throughout the day and night. Staff typically recognise and characterise MAU as 'chaotic', with working on one seen as a badge of honour, second only to the emergency department (in the UK, the Accident and Emergency Unit (A&E) itself). These units are not areas designed or conducive to supporting the needs of any particular patient group, which means they can be particularly disorientating for the large number of people living with dementia admitted to them. Prior to fieldwork, our network of carers and their partners living with dementia all told us they had poor experiences of this setting and found it a 'frightening' place.

In total, during our first phase of fieldwork within 5 hospitals (which represents our first funded ethnography), we spent 155 days within these wards, observing everyday cultures of care and the ways in which care was organised and delivered at the bedside for people living with dementia. We focussed on the work of nurses and healthcare assistants, following ward teams from handover and shadowing individuals as they worked at the bedside. We watched these teams throughout the day, at evenings, through night shifts and across weekends. We also followed other members of staff who entered these wards sporadically, those arriving to conduct certain tasks or see specific patients. During this time, we carried out 486 ethnographic interviews with staff, carers, and, importantly, patients living with dementia themselves. A further cohort of people living with dementia and their families were followed during and after their admission.

We were still wandering these wards (within three further hospitals) at the time of writing (this began in October 2018 and continued until October 2019) and we also draw on these data in this book. We do not quote directly from the data collected from these wards in this book, but the phenomena we describe here were repeated and reinforced across the later wards. While looking at other elements of everyday care we observed the same patterns of behaviour from both people living with dementia and the staff caring for them, the drive to support them and the organisational obstacles that prevent this, and echoes of the deeply engrained ward cultures which exist from site to site. While collecting these data we also increasingly utilised visual and participatory methods to involve a wider group of people living with dementia, their carers and their families, input from which we directly draw on within this book.

Ethnography by its very nature is incomplete and yet we do not have the space to do justice to all our data and analysis here. Given the significant and growing body of literature within the fields of social psychology, nursing, sociology, and anthropology focussing on the lived experience of people living with dementia and their carers and family members, within this book, we largely draw on our observational data within the over 600,000 words of fieldnotes, taken between 2015 and 2017, with a smaller number taken from the 2018–2019 fieldnotes (700,000 words) in order to examine ward cultures, which remain relatively underexamined but critical in informing the care of people living with dementia.

The ethics of entering these wards

Conducting any type of research within hospital settings in the UK requires NHS ethics committee screening, governance, and permissions, an important and necessary process, but which is a source of 'mock terror' in the corridors of universities across the UK. It was only once we had secured funding and started to uncover and identify the many stages of these (rightly) rigorous and complex governance processes that the barriers to ethnographic research (and research more widely) within hospital wards started to become clear to us and to become a pressing concern.

We had been through these processes and obtained NHS ethics committee approvals for previous ethnographic research examining out-patient clinics. However, these studies had examined highly specialised fields of medicine and healthcare (e.g. clinical genetics services). This meant that they constituted naturally bounded and distinct entities, containing within them a limited and known group of participants consisting of small clinical teams, out-patients and their families (these clinics also had a narrow focus on diagnosing and classifying a range of rare familial and de-novo genetic conditions (Featherstone et al. 2005, 2006)). In contrast, we could see there were some particular challenges in developing rigorous procedures for our hospital ethnography. We could foresee that asking for permission to observe everyday care in the busy and high-pressured context of hospital wards, where the teams and individuals entering them cannot be predicted or controlled, and involving people living with dementia during their acute hospital admission, would all require sensitive and nuanced approaches. While we found our NHS ethics committee supportive with regards to the study in itself, it took two hearings with the committee, and significant modifications to the protocol and the study documentation, before the committee was satisfied the study posed no risk for patients and staff, a process that took close to six months.

What we learnt quickly was that what made complete sense on paper, and in discussion with a research committee, in a pleasant air-conditioned conference room in a non-descript business hotel at a motorway junction, did not translate to the constant motion of an acute ward. In particular, obtaining written consent prior to all observations was not very practical within the fast pace of these wards. Staff were always busy, and patients could be sleeping or too unwell to approach at the start of a shift. Following initial fieldwork within two wards at our first hospital, we returned to the committee to ask for amendments to the study protocol. A system of obtaining initial verbal consent was agreed to minimise interruptions to staff at busy points in their shifts, such as handovers at the start of shifts, with formal written consent taken later for those directly observed or spoken to during the study. This modification was also supported by the ward teams, who said that looking back, they appreciated being able to gain a clearer understanding of the unfamiliar research method and the type of data we were collecting once fieldwork had started.

We also found that the use of the formal detailed consent forms required and approved by the committee were often difficult for people living with dementia during their admission. This is not surprising given that they were all admitted for a suspected acute condition such as an infection within MAU, or a fracture, and most likely a hip replacement within the Trauma and Orthopaedics (T&O) wards. With the support of the NHS ethics committee, we agreed that all patients would be informed of the study and the research at the start of and during all periods of observations, when we would also emphasise that they were able to choose to opt out then or at any point during the observations. We used a form of process consent (Dewing 2007) and spoke to each individual patient in the area of observation throughout the periods of observation to regularly re-introduce ourselves in order to familiarise and remind them of who we were, our role, the study and what it involved, and to request their consent verbally throughout the periods of observation. The committee agreed that patients within the ward would only be required to sign a consent form if they were approached to take part in interviews or if the researcher closely observed the care they received at their bedside.

We took this time obtaining and refining our approaches to consent as an opportunity to develop our understandings of and impacts of dementia by attending undergraduate nursing modules on dementia care, shadowing clinical staff, including an experienced dementia care specialist nurse, and became 'dementia friends' by completing the online UK Alzheimer's Society awareness course. We also spent time with people living with dementia, carers, and families, through our local networks. We wanted to ensure we reflected the right approaches in being with and supporting people living with dementia so that they could make decisions about taking part in the research and were given opportunities to express and share their experiences.

We are grateful to the members of NHS Research Ethics Service, and in particular the members of the Wales Research Ethics Committee, not only for approving our studies but also for their advice and critique of our study designs and approaches to involvement. Their knowledge of the wards was invaluable in shaping our project into something that was both workable within the ward setting, protecting the participants within it, and for meeting the requirements of the Mental Capacity Act 2005 (Section 31). With their help and feedback our initial study was approved in June 2015 (15/WA/0191) and subsequently accepted by NHS Research Permissions Wales (and subsequently the newly formed Health Research Authority), with whom recruitment for our studies has been managed and recorded via their Central Portfolio Management System. Amendments were approved for our observations in December 2015, to improve our consent and recruitment processes to better fit the realities of life within these wards. Approval for our ongoing second study was again granted by members of the Wales Research Ethics Committee in April 2018 (18/WA/0033), and accepted by the Health Research Authority and Health and Care Research Wales in September 2018.

All sites, individuals, and data collected were anonymised and sorted in line with the Data Protection Act 1998, and NHS England Data Protection Policy 2014. In order to protect the anonymity of our participants, all patients directly presented within this book have been given a pseudonym, and any recognisable features of individuals, wards, or sites have been altered or removed. Staff are referred to only by their role or job title, and the generic term for each role is used to prevent revealing participating individuals, wards, and hospitals. This reflects our recording practices to ensure participant anonymity (patients and staff) within our fieldnotes, which was to refer to patients by their bed number and staff by their role. Although this reflects a familiar practice within these wards, we are aware that it also has the potential to be dehumanising and desensitising.

Similarly, when we discuss 'these wards', it is an amalgamation. This amalgamation was straightforward in many ways: with only minor exceptions, the overall cultures of these wards, and the organisation and delivery of care within them, were surprisingly similar and comparable. These hospitals have also been anonymised. We considered replicating the strategy of Julius Roth, and the ethnographies of the 1950s and 1960s, who in part inspired our work and this book, and giving each site a pseudonym, but have settled instead on giving each site a simple alphabetic code to maintain the anonymity of these wards and the participants who supported our research.

Beyond protecting anonymity, the safety of all participants within our ethnography was a key priority for us. Before undertaking this study, the ethics of observing care, and the ethics of reporting (where necessary) what we observed, was frequently discussed with staff in the hospital sites and with our carers' steering group. In meetings with the NHS REC that approved our study it was clarified that although we technically did not have a clinical duty of care (both researchers were academics without clinical qualifications or professional affiliations), we would still be bound to safeguard any patient participants observed over the course of our ethnography.

Before starting our ethnography, we undertook (and have since updated) Good Clinical Practice certification, Adult Safeguarding certification, and Protection of Vulnerable Adults (POVA) training. We were made aware of safeguarding and whistleblowing procedures at each site and had a named member of staff (the site principal investigator or research nurse on shift) to contact if malpractice or behaviour that put vulnerable people at risk was observed.

Over the course of our ethnography, as will be detailed in the course of this book, we saw many aspects of everyday practice that concerned us, but were both viewed and described as normal practice within these wards and were not considered problematic. The examples we present throughout this book were not isolated and we have taken care not to include any atypical or unusual examples from our data. Each formed part of the systemic and established everyday routine practice within every ward at each hospital site. While some of the phenomena presented and discussed in this book may be upsetting, over the course of our fieldwork we did not witness malicious behaviour or isolated incidents of deviance that placed a patient at risk. Instead, we observed how the everyday organisation and delivery of bedside care itself often has the potential to place individual and cohorts of patients at risk, but that this is part of the routine and established cultures of these hospitals and reflected the everyday care practices within these wards. At no point did we feel that any individual member of staff or ward team was acting in a way that required escalation or whistleblowing. Had we observed behaviour that we felt breached guidelines, or deliberately placed a patient in danger, we would have immediately ceased observations and reported the incident in line with site procedures. Throughout our time within the wards, and during our research, we regularly presented emerging finding and our analysis to our wider research team, steering groups and collaborators, including nurses, allied health professionals, clinicians, and NHS Trust leads. Although it was agreed that the care observed could be detrimental or distressing to a person living with dementia, it was also routine and recognisable to them as the everyday practices of staff within acute wards.

We did, however, question staff about their practises and frequently intervened to support people living with dementia and their families and carers where we felt it was necessary to protect and support the comfort of the patient. People living with dementia would tell us frequently that they wanted to go to the bathroom or that they were in pain, or shared their concerns (about their home, their family or their pets, or how to pay for their care). In response to these disclosures, we (with permission from the patient) would inform ward staff and ensure that this was not forgotten and was attended to by the ward team.

In addition, we were sometimes the only member of 'staff' spending uninterrupted time on a hospital bay and so would regularly ask patients if they needed anything. Sometimes when staff were not present or able to be called quickly to a bay, we provided immediate support and help. For example, if we observed a patient trying to get out of bed unaided, leaving the ward, or putting themselves at immediate risk of physical danger, we would call staff and, if necessary, intervene. Similarly, we would fetch cups of tea and pour glasses of water and carry out other simple requests within these wards when required. Although we accept that this may have, on occasion, contaminated the purity of the research, the welfare of those within these wards was always our priority.

Notes on our use of language

The reader may have already noticed the regular use of the phrase 'people living with dementia' within this preface and we continue this throughout the book. Similarly, we refer to 'people' rather than 'patients' wherever possible because we believe the use of 'patients' reduces personhood. Viewing people within these wards as nothing more than a patient increases the potential for dehumanisation. This and similar phrases are used following discussions with people living with dementia and carers, and in order to follow the recommendation of DEEP (Dementia Engagement and Empowerment Project, a UK network of groups of people living with dementia), a UK charitable organisation which promotes the empowerment of and engagement with people living with dementia (https://www.dementiavoices.org.uk). It is crucial to remember that the experiences detailed within this book are experienced by *people* who are also living with a condition. Similarly, we hope never to promote the use of dehumanising language and will never use words such as 'sufferer', 'burden' and other descriptors that have contributed historically to the inequalities experienced by people living with dementia.

Throughout this book we also refer to 'dementia'. We recognise that this is a simplistic representation of a more complex constellation of conditions (which we will discuss in more detail later in this book) and we do so in order to reflect everyday usage within these wards, and because it represents everyday current usage in England and Wales. Later in this book we discuss the issues surrounding the classification of dementia, and the recognition, and attribution of this condition in the person within these wards in more detail.

At the same time, we do at points in this book make reference to some terms that contradict and are at odds with these guidelines. We choose these words carefully, and with much thought, recognising that they are both evocative and discomfiting, but that their use is important if we are to reflect the world of these wards and their impacts on the people within them. This means that we will at times describe behaviours of people living with dementia viewed by ward staff as 'disruptive', 'inappropriate', 'transgressive' and as 'resistance' and 'refusal' to care. We will highlight people being described by staff within these wards as 'challenging', 'agitated', 'aggressive', and 'confused', who are 'wandering' instead of walking, who require 'toileting' instead of a person who needs support with continence needs, or requiring 'feeding' instead of requiring support to eat a meal. We do not, however, condone this language. This is the language of these wards and the wider cultures of these hospitals. These terms reflect how the phenomena we witnessed was recognised, conceptualised, understood, and articulated by the many social actors within it.

The understandings found within these wards also reflect the conceptualisations of dementia and the behaviour of people living with dementia found within the wider biomedical literature. They have been recognised clinically as part of a constellation of 'neuropsychiatric symptoms' commonly described as 'behavioural and psychological symptoms' (BPSD) associated with dementia.

Importantly, a re-evaluation of and debates about the appropriateness of these terms is ongoing (Wolverson et al. 2019), to reflect perspectives that emphasise the importance of the social and clinical contexts in which they occur and that these 'symptoms' may reflect the communication of unmet need (Cohen-Mansfield and Mintzer 2005) and as such are currently being reframed, for example, as 'behavioural expressions' (Macaulay 2018) and 'stress and distress' (Wolverson et al. 2019) as more closely reflecting the experiences of people living with dementia. We support interpretations which see these 'behaviours' as reflecting an individual's responses to the ways in which care is organised and delivered to them at their bedside and the difficulties people living with dementia may have in communicating their needs verbally (and promptly to meet the expected pace of care) within the acute setting (Featherstone et al. 2019).

The representation of vulnerable people

Many of the events we have observed during the course of this ethnography have had a profound impact on us and undoubtedly are deeply troubling, distressing, and disturbing. However, we do not present these stories to provide a voyeuristic insight into the pain and distress of vulnerable people or to shame and blame the typically low-paid, overworked, and often-powerless frontline staff. Instead, our goal is to reveal this hidden world, to make the experiences and humanity of everyone, of all the people (patients and staff) within these wards visible and to make known the high stakes of these invisibilities for everyone.

None of the events and examples we present within this monograph are exceptional, unique, or unusual, but instead are chosen carefully to represent everyday patterns of ward organisation and cultures of care that were present and observable across our ethnographic data set as ordinary and mundane practice within the many acute wards we spent time in. Additional layers of powerlessness and precariousness were created and brought into being once a person became recognised as also living with dementia within these wards.

Note

1 In the England this is the role of the Care Quality Commission (CQC). As an independent regulator, the CQC monitor and inspect hospitals to ensure they meet fundamental standards of quality and safety. Hospitals can be classed as 'outstanding' if assessed to be giving exceptional care, or 'failing' or in 'special measures' when performing badly.

Acknowledgements

We would not have reached this point in our research without the extraordinary support, advice, commitment, and friendship, of our carers' steering group. Their involvement was, and continues to be, vital in highlighting the acute setting as a key area of urgent need, shaping our research agenda. They and their partners have continued to support us throughout our project, commenting on the appropriateness of our methods, discussing and debating our analysis and findings. We particularly thank Rosie Tope, Jackie Askey, Anne Davies, Peggy Martin, Viv Morgan, Julie Stacey, Betty Roderick, David Jones, Lynne Jeffrey, Chris Jones, Joan Gabe-Jenkin, and all the members of the Carers' steering group for all their support and for keeping us focussed on our goal of using sociology to understanding everyday cultures of care and to improve the quality and humanity of care people living with dementia receive during an acute hospital admission. We also remember George Askey, whose experiences continue to inform our work.

None of this could have happened without the support of the National Institute of Health Research Health Services and Delivery Research (NIHR HS&DR) funding programme. They funded our hospital ethnography through two consecutive studies 'The management of refusal of food, drink and medications by people with dementia admitted to hospital with an acute condition' (project number 13/10/80) and 'Understanding how to facilitate continence for people living with dementia in acute hospital settings: raising awareness and improving care' (project number 15/136/67). We particularly want to acknowledge and thank Avril Lloyd and Nick Eaton for their support and kindness as our NIHR Monitoring Research Managers, for always being there as we navigated the more complex governance and administrative hurdles and through the highs and lows that are inevitably part of any research. We would also like to acknowledge the support of the larger NIHR team and the reviewers of our research proposals and reports for improving the rigour of our research and for their support. The views and opinions expressed therein are those of the authors and do not necessarily reflect those of the HS&DR researcher-led funding stream, NIHR, the NHS or the Department of Health.

We are, of course, extremely grateful to all the people living with dementia, their families and carers, and the nurses, healthcare assistants, and the medical teams, who have shared their stories, supported our work, and given us the encouragement to use our ethnography to improve care for people living with dementia, and to improve the working lives of nurses and healthcare assistants working in the acute setting. We would like to acknowledge them all individually; but are required to preserve their anonymity.

It would be a misconception to think that our research within this book simply involved the two of us travelling the country armed only with a bag full of note pads and pens (although that was a key element). It would not be possible without wider collaboration, supporting, guiding, and reflecting on the research. The work presented in this book, and indeed our ongoing research in this area, would not be possible without the wisdom, patience, and friendship of Jane Harden, Paula Boddington, Sonia Vougioukalou, Jane Hopkinson and Amanda King from the School of Healthcare Sciences at Cardiff University, Karen Harrison Dening, Head of Research and Publications at Dementia UK and Jackie Bridges from the School of Healthcare Sciences at University of Southampton. We would also like to thank our External Oversight Group, for incredibly stimulating and encouraging meetings: Chris Roberts (activist and living with dementia), Jayne Goodrick (activist and carer), Lorraine Edmunds (Dementia Strategy, Welsh Government), Alexandra Feast (University College London), Paula Saukko (Loughborough University), John Vorhaus (University College London), Laura Cole (King's College London), Chris Chatterton (academic and activist), as well as the many academics, activists, and clinicians who have supported and provided feedback on our research at conferences and symposia over the last five years.

We would also like to thank our many colleagues, mentors, and friends who support our work: Paul Atkinson (who taught us all we know about ethnography), Kathy Rowan (for imparting the skills or 'sport' of grant writing), Sue Bale (for helping us to navigate governance and for introducing us to the world of the wards), and Andrew Scott (for his transformative coaching).

We are relative newcomers to the field of 'dementia' and we have found the research networks within it have been incredibly supportive. We would particularly like to acknowledge Esme Moniz-Cook, Jem Bhatt, Georgina Charlesworth, Rowan Harwood, and Martin Orrell, and the members of interdem.org, a pan-European network of researchers collaborating in research aimed at improving the quality of life of people with dementia and their supporters, across Europe.

We have drawn on a wide range of expertise in not only delivering our research, but also finding ways to communicate to as large and diverse an audience as possible through a variety of media. Special thanks go to Nick Daw, for his work as Director of Photography and for producing, shooting, and editing our short films. To Dawn Driscoll (Dawn Driscoll PR) for her strategy and delivery of our knowledge transfer programme, Tyler Chambers for strategy, mentoring, and managing our social media, to Sophie Nightingale, for our beautiful branding and illustrations, and to Chris Hartwill (Director), and Kelly Hewitt (Producer) for their support in filming the stories that accompany this research.

We are also indebted to the teams at Chapter Arts Centre, Cardiff and to Film Hub Wales, who all share our commitment to increasing access to the arts and using film to reduce social isolation. They have always been enthusiastic about collaborating with us to improve access to the arts and film for people living with dementia and their families: Sally Griffith, Claire Vaughan, Ellie Russell, Hana Lewis, Lisa Nesbitt, and Toki Allinson.

All of these contributors supported the research that underpins this book, giving up their time with the goal of improving the care people living with dementia experience in hospital. With their support we were able to embed ourselves in hospital wards across England and Wales.

Our programme continues beyond the publication of this book. The frequently updated results of our wider research programme, our research reports, consultation events, and education and training courses to support ward staff, along with short films featuring our collaborators; people living with dementia, their family carers, and the nursing staff that care for them, can be viewed at our website, www.storiesofdementia.com, along with updates on our ongoing projects and future work.

1 Ward cultures of care

Early in our observations, a Senior House Officer (SHO) from the Trauma and Orthopaedic department invited us to leave these wards and wander the wider hospital with him. It is his Friday night on-call shift. 'Bring your notebook!', he instructs. It was already dark. Outside, in the town centre that flanks the outskirts of the hospital, the shops had already closed and the bars were starting to fill up. Walking past the bank of waiting ambulances and the huddle of smokers in dressing gowns and slippers, following a trail of cigarette stubs, we meet him in the small public entrance at the side of the main building leading towards A&E. We follow him up to the third floor and he swipes us through an unmarked door to the backstage of the hospital. The main public corridors are brightly lit and starkly institutional, but this very long corridor is poorly lit and feels unloved. After a few turns, we arrive at the very shabby and harshly lit on-call room. Threadbare and frayed swivel chairs are lined up in front of a bank of old computers, each linked to multiple screens. To one side the large windows face out onto the small atrium, with the other wall a bank of whiteboards listing the surgical schedule. The two Registrars are already there, along with the SHO from the day shift, ready for 'handover' and the chance to go home. Once this is complete and the night shift SHO has the handover list (a very basic printout of key patient details - name, hospital number, and location) and pager (most hospitals still use pagers, commonly referred to as 'the bleep'), we head back out... 'BLEEP', to the paediatric ward to check on a young boy with a fractured arm. His parents are frustrated at the length of time taken over his admission, and the SHO explains the concerns about potential swelling and the importance of monitoring his arm... 'BLEEP', into the surgical assessment unit to meet a man in his 50s who had been covering his ulcerated toe with sticking plaster. It may need amputating... 'BLEEP', into 'minors' (the minor injury unit is the part of the emergency department that treats urgent, but not life-threatening injuries and is often called the walk-in, urgent care, or urgent treatment centre) to meet a young woman experiencing numbness in her arm and a woman in her 40s whose fingers had been trapped in a sun lounger... 'BLEEP', next door to A&E, where we arrive at cubicle 19 to meet June who is living with dementia.

> It is midnight and June is alone in the cubicle. She is clearly in a lot of pain, and extremely distressed. She is a tiny woman with pale skin and soft silver-grey hair, and her very large beautiful blue-grey eyes are unblinking,

> staring up at the bright lights overhead. She looks rigid, almost locked in a twisted position on the trolley and appears terrified. No one from the care home where she lives came with her in the ambulance and the two very tall medics standing over her are calling her by the wrong name (the A&E team continue to do this throughout the night).

June is one of the many people who make up one of the most significant patient populations in our hospitals. A key contemporary transformation is the increasing numbers of people living with dementia within our hospitals, with their care constituting an increasingly significant part of the everyday work.

Globally, the hospital has become a key site of care for people living with dementia, who are now estimated to represent up to 63.0% of the acute population (Mukadam and Sampson 2011). In the UK, at least one in four acute hospital beds will be occupied by a person living with dementia at any given time (Alzheimer's Society 2009, 2016), the equivalent of 3.2 million bed days per year. However, the Department of Health now recognise that these figures may be underestimates, with some hospitals reporting this patient group represents as much as 50% of their acute admissions (Alzheimer's Society 2016).

> As June lies on the trolley, the attending team tell us she is a '90 year old lady living in a nursing home, right NoF (Neck of Femur or hip joint) with a background of dementia, a subcapital fracture' (a common fracture that extends through the head and neck of the femur). He reads from the file: 'She is steady with the Zimmer, she is a healthy 90-year-old, only dementia, nothing else.' The senior supervises and talks the junior through 'doing a block' (a Fascia iliaca compartment block - a local anesthetic for the pain) before they send her for further X-rays. The Registrar gets the sterile pack for the block procedure for him. 'We are aiming for femoral nerve cover and it's important to check the blood pressure every fifteen minutes. What will the patient complain of?'
>
> His junior responds. 'Numbness of mouth.'
>
> 'Yes, but she won't because she is pretty out of it. You will never get full sterility because it's the groin, but you don't want to add bugs to that area.'
>
> The junior pulls on a pair of disposable gloves, takes the needle and hovers over her hip.
>
> 'Find your landmarks again, stay still (to the patient who he is still calling by the wrong name) you will feel a sharp scratch, this is to numb the area for the big needle' then to the junior 'so give it 30 seconds to work, often people go straight in with the second, but this defeats the purpose.'
>
> June interrupts to tell them 'I feel sick.'
>
> 'Don't worry June, if you feel sick here is a bowl.' The senior smiles at her and stands at her side, placing a bowl on her chest, near to her mouth. He holds it for her and watches the junior. 'Make sure you are comfortable, take your time, once you are through the skin come back.'

The junior pulls back and the needle is just under the thin pale skin of the hip. 'Come back through the skin and then the first pop and the second pop through the fascia, in thin frail people it can be difficult to identify, so just do it again. Withdraw and do it again … '

The junior does this: 'Yes, I felt the first and second pop.'

'... and inject. It should go in reasonably freely.'

He is still holding the bowl for June.

'Are you still feeling a bit sick darling or are you OK? All done there madam. How are you feeling, June? It should start feeling better.'

People living with dementia are not admitted because of their dementia diagnosis, but because they require an unscheduled emergency admission, typically due to a physical injury such as a hip fracture (as in June's case), head injury, urinary tract infection, pneumonia, or a lower respiratory infection and therefore need to be admitted and treated within a specialist acute ward. Conversely, people living with dementia admitted for assessment are frequently found to have no clinical reason for their admission. For a person without dementia, this would be the point of discharge. For a person living with dementia, however, this will typically initiate a pattern of further assessment, extending their admission. These patterns were reflected in the patient populations and their admitting conditions in the acute wards within our study and more widely during our visits to many other hospitals in England and Wales over the last six years.

June is curled up on the trolley partly covered in a thin blanket and is clinging tightly onto the raised metal bed rail. I now notice that she has been clutching her false teeth tightly in her other hand all this time, the sick bowl resting on her chest. The medical team move to the workstations at the centre of the unit and I go over to her and hold her hand. She tells me 'I am in terrible pain'.

I tell the Registrar and he leans over so he is hovering slightly above her head, looking down into her eyes: 'Hello June, are you in pain?'

'Terrible.'

'Where?'

She moves her hand to the side of her stomach.

'Can you remember at all what happened to you?'

'No.'

'June, do you know where you are now? How much does it hurt on a scale of 1 to 10?'

To me he turns and explains. 'She is not oriented to place, it's hard to get a history because she is not compos mentis.'

He turns back to June 'Do you know where you are, sweetheart?'

People living with dementia are a highly vulnerable group within the acute hospital setting; they are at higher risk of delayed discharge, and likely to experience functional decline during their admission (Mukadam and Sampson 2011). They also have a markedly higher short-term mortality (Care Quality Commission 2014), with almost a quarter dying during admission (Sampson et al. 2009). Dementia is a progressive and life-limiting condition, and so on the surface these high rates can, and typically are, viewed as 'natural' and to some extent inevitable, following an admission. These facts appear unremarkable and to be expected. They are attributed to their dementia, which is currently the leading cause of death in England and Wales (Office of National Statistics 2019). But what if the cultures of care, the low expectations of recovery, the ways in which care is organised and delivered to people living with dementia within this setting was significant? What if hospital care itself contributes to these high rates? Public enquiries have repeatedly identified unacceptable quality and humanity of care (Care Quality Commission 2011, 2014), including the widespread and systemic deprivation of dignity and respect (Francis report 2013), raise serious concerns about the cultures of care for people living with dementia (Andrews report 2014) and their consequences. What if these cultures of care are contributing to the acceleration of decline and death within this population, and making what is unnatural seem nothing more than a natural and inevitable progression?

> The bleep called us away to another patient in a different part of the hospital. When we return to A&E to see June, she looks much more comfortable and alert. She is lying propped up in the bed, she has an IV drip in her arm, a mobile monitoring unit attached by a clip to her finger, and is still holding her false teeth in her left hand. The Junior stands next to her at the bedside and bends down over her, close to her face and raises his voice:
>
> 'YOU. ARE. IN. HOSPITAL.'
>
> 'I am in hospital. I fell down', she responds.
>
> 'You have a fracture in your left hip [it is her right hip which is fractured] so we will fix it.'
>
> 'Can you?', she says, looking pleadingly up into his eyes.
>
> 'Yes, they will do a hip replacement and that way it will be fixed – if we don't do the operation it will take a very long time to heal.'
>
> 'Yes, you are very, very kind.' June has a very soft and gentle tremulous voice.
>
> As we are about to leave, she calls me over and holds onto my arm: 'Don't go away, I have a pain in my stomach, it's a nasty pain in my stomach (she seems to really consider what the pain is and places a powerful emphasis on 'nasty'), it's there (she lifts the sheets and points to her side of her body), it's a nasty pain, I am afraid to move … it's awful pain, it's terrible pain.'
>
> The junior responds to this. 'We have your morphine and that can sometimes make you feel a bit sick. We will give you something for the pain. Can I discuss the operation? I am going to mark it.' The junior takes a black marker pen and marks her hip.
>
> 'It's a sharp nasty pain.' Again she places real emphasis on 'nasty', pointing to her side. As he fills in the paperwork at the bedside he tells me. 'She needs morphine, as much as needed because of her NoF.' I hold her hand.
>
> June says 'Don't leave me. I am in awful pain, I am in terrible pain, Don't go away.'

'We are calling your family and getting you up to a hospital bed and you will have surgery. We will give you some pain medicine, IV paracetamol, and we will send you up', responds the SHO.

We find it extremely upsetting to leave her as the next bleep on the pager calls us away. She looks extremely vulnerable. It is 4 a.m.

June's admission also demonstrates the narrow understandings and expectations of a person living with dementia, the restricted repertoire of talk directed at them, and the impact it has on the person within these wards. Despite June giving detailed descriptions of her pain, the senior member of the medical team describes her as 'not compos mentis' [sic]. Throughout our time in these wards we repeatedly heard the loud and slowly enunciated phrase 'YOU. ARE. IN. HOSPITAL.' directed at people living with dementia (by staff across all roles, specialisms, and grades).

This trope was a typical opening line when greeting or responding to a patient living with dementia, particularly when the person seemed anxious, afraid, or distressed (as was the case with June above). Its ubiquity was unquestioned, it was an everyday part of these cultures of care, even though such approaches typically appeared to generate further distress and fear in the patient being addressed. This is the everyday work at the bedside. Importantly, this also indicates the systematic failure of these institutional cultures to consider how best to organise and deliver care that meets the needs of this significant population or to provide meaningful support and training for staff within these wards in caring for them.

Cultures of care and their consequences

The hospital is a place set apart, but the social world of the wards within it reflect the wider social inequalities and invisibilities people living with dementia experience every day. Hospitals have often been described as separate from everyday life. Coser describes the hospital as a 'tight little island' (1962: 3), where the patient is 'cut adrift' (1962: 39) from the world. Goffman suggests hospital wards are 'little islands of vivid, encapturing activity' ([1961] 1991: 68) within the total institution. By contrast, others have described the hospital as more closely reflecting the wider social world, 'a small society' (Caudill 1958: 3), with Roth and Eddy concluding it is 'society in miniature' (1967: 19). We too found that these wards were a place set apart, but also one that powerfully reflected wider social values. The hospital ward is thus a site which has its own culture, 'rules' that must be understood and learnt by all those entering it, but also where wider cultural understandings of dementia persist.

In the care of people living with dementia, 'this question of the culture in a hospital is absolutely crucial' (House of Lords House of Commons Joint Committee on Human Rights 2006–2007: 44). A detailed examination of these cultures of care, 'the way things are (actually) done around here' (Drennan 1992), and their impacts on people living with dementia is required if we are to understand and improve care outcomes. Yet such impacts were rarely considered by these organisations or by the teams caring for them within these wards. 'Symptoms' attributed to dementia that ward staff (and the wider hospital organisation) viewed as the most problematic (this included resistance to timetabled care, and behaviour viewed as disruptive, inappropriate, or transgressive) were behaviours that did not easily fit within or recognise the rules of these wards. These 'symptoms' were extremely common – for example every person living with dementia we observed within our study resisted or refused care at some point during our observations, yet these responses were always located within the individual and attributed to their diagnosis of dementia. It was as if the person living with dementia was 'cut adrift' on an island within these wards, viewed as a person defined essentially by their condition, existing in isolation, and as if unaffected by the social world in which they find themselves. Rarely, if ever, was there any consideration that many of these responses could in fact be caused by the ward environment, a reaction to the organisation and timetabled delivery of routine bedside care, and care practices within these wards. Understanding the impacts of ward cultures in shaping these interactions and their consequences is critical if we are to improve the quality and humanity of care received by people living with dementia receive and also to support the staff caring for them (Digby et al. 2017) within this key site of care.

Cultures of attribution

Within this book we explore the ways in which *dementia* as a condition is recognised and attributed in the everyday work of these wards. Dementia was ascribed to individuals by ward staff through acts of recognition; their identification and differentiation of a limited number of specific classificatory features. Importantly, within these wards, this was a taken-for-granted diagnostic category, a routine and everyday practice of naming and claiming applied to large numbers of older people. An unremarkable and consistent feature of bedside work was the repeated querying and testing of memory, that cast doubt on the mental acuity of all older people within these wards: 'to ask about the minds of old people is essential and expected'(Cohen 1998: 16), with an expectation that a deficit would be identified. We will explore these practices, their powerful consequences, and the ways this informed the cultures of care within these wards within Chapter 4.

Ward staff focused starkly on the cognitive features associated with the condition, primarily on identifying memory loss in the abstract. Cognition was always understood linguistically, and all assessments of the person focused on judgements of their interaction with staff and the ability to respond and express themselves (for example, by demonstrating reason) verbally. This became evident at the bedside in the preoccupation with assessing a person's ability to recall personal details (typically their date of birth and age), general knowledge (with an emphasis on facts about the British monarchy, such as 'Who is the Queen of England?'), historical dates (typically focused on the world wars), and testing the person's memory in the context of the now ('What time is it?'), repeatedly prompting and requiring verbal confirmation of whether the person knew they were in a hospital, why they were in the hospital, or where the hospital was. Non-verbal, or embodied, communication was not recognised as such, but understood and viewed by staff as resistive, disruptive, inappropriate, or transgressive behaviour to be managed and limited within these wards. Such approaches effaced the complexity of the category, the range of symptoms associated with the condition,[1] and the wide array of potential impacts on the person. Importantly, these understandings could have significant longer-term consequences for the person, informing judgements of their cognitive capacity and their ability to make decisions about their care, expectations of recovery, and place of discharge (whether they could go back home).

The category 'dementia' also appeared to be a default category applied to a far larger social cluster, to include the wider population of older patients within these wards, a process Zerubavel (1996) terms 'lumping'. For the significant group of older people within these wards, symptoms that could be associated with their admitting condition (for example, older people admitted with an infection or delirium can present with confusion, disorientation, agitation) or the impact of the ward environment itself (as we have described above), could potentially become recognised and interpreted as behavioural features of dementia as a condition, and this categorisation could quickly become applied informally by ward staff to the person. Importantly, unlike most other conditions, dementia, and the signage and symbols used to represent it within these wards, created a label that could become attached to individual patients during bedside care and informal staff exchanges during shifts, and interact with and enter recording practices. An assumed (mis)diagnosis by non-expert staff within these wards could quickly transform into an effective diagnosis in the delivery of everyday practice at the bedside.

Such practices had significant consequences at the bedside, including reducing opportunities to see any other potential underlying cause in the individual, such as possibly representing a different underlying pathology, an urgent personal care need, or experiences of fear and distress associated with the admission itself. We identified processes of contagion and spread in the recognition and application of this category. The established routine care practices believed to be appropriate for one group – people living with dementia – could quickly become attached to a wider group of older people within these wards. This could be exacerbated by common practices of zoning or 'corralling' patients who share specific attributes placed together within wards and bays. The organisational practice of assigning beds by dependency (Roth and Eddy 1967) or to 'age grade' patients (Zerubavel 1979) within wards is a long-standing one. Often this resulted in older people living both with and without dementia being treated alongside one another in the bays and areas of these wards. Within clinical medicine, the classification of the 'elderly' or 'older' patient and its association with pathology emerged as part of the development of geriatric medicine in the 19th Century (Kirk 1992) and continues to be debated (Zhavoronkov and Bhullar 2015). The classification of the older patient within the contemporary hospital is 65 years old and over, with a further category of 'old old' at 75 and 'oldest old' for patients who are 85 years and older (Wise 2010). Thus, the routine interactional practices and bedside care believed to be appropriate for people living with dementia could quickly become recognised and applied as standard care for a large and heterogeneous group of patients aged 65 years and over, but who were understood within these wards to be a homogeneous population with similar care needs.

Institutional, administrative, and ward practices reflect and reinforce these reductive understandings and recognition of categories. This was visible in the everyday naming and labelling practices that pervaded both the everyday talk and within the documentation used by ward teams. Informal categories, including 'climbers', 'feeders' and 'shouters', were coupled with institutionalised terms that transformed the meanings of everyday behaviour. Walking within these wards was universally understood as being without purpose and described as 'wandering' (hence the title of this book), a person asking or expressing the desire to go home or trying to leave the ward was referred to as 'absconding'. To be assessed as physically able get out of bed was to be 'mobilised' or 'self-mobilising', with any independent actions becoming 'self-care' or the individual being described as 'self-caring'. These were mixed with the broad 'catch-all' categories of recognition such as 'confusion', 'pleasantly confused', the 'muddled', and a wider range of prodromal versions of the condition attributed to the person through the use of queries such as '?dementia' or 'suspected dementia' assigned to large numbers of individuals by non-specialist staff.

This everyday terminology existed alongside an array of signage and images representing dementia that proliferated these wards, becoming attached to individuals via admission and bedside boards that highlight attention to the idea of dementia in the person. On walking through the main corridor intersecting any ward, at the nursing station, on noticeboards, on toilet doors, one will witness a myriad of magnets, laminated signs, symbols, and handwritten abbreviations, all representing dementia. We found the widespread use of signage and symbols placed at the bedside typically took the form of either a blue butterfly or a blue flower (forget-me-not), but we observed many more, to signify to the ward that the person at that bedside has a diagnosis of dementia. Within Chapter 3, we explore the prominent use of signage to classify people living with dementia, and the ways they powerfully informed the expectations of not only how these patients should be cared for, but where they should be cared for (almost always somewhere else).

These labels could all manifest during the shift handover, during interdisciplinary rounds and meetings, and in informal talk within the ward team, which could quickly solidify as a taken-for-granted diagnosis. These practices reflect dementia as a public condition; all classes and types of non-specialist staff had the right to recognise, adjudicate, name, or (in some cases) dismiss a diagnosis of dementia. Because of this, the hospital ward is a place where a dementia diagnosis could fluctuate; it could be applied, removed, and denied for a person. While dementia remains an incurable degenerative neurocognitive disorder, the practices of its application within an acute ward means a person may 'have dementia' for the duration of a shift, until a transfer, or until discharge. Within these wards dementia was a very public condition, but it was also a diagnosis that was rarely, if ever, shared or discussed directly with the person.

Cultures of care and institutional 'looping'

Importantly, we found powerful interactions between the ways in which care was organised and delivered at the bedside and the ways in which patients living with dementia responded and reacted to care. The repeated cycles of highly structured care practices at the bedside (which we will explore in detail within Chapters 5, 6, and 7), in turn, amplified both the person's distress and the care practices used by staff in response to what they viewed as the 'behavioural' features of their dementia. We identified that these understandings typically prompted a tightening of the timetables of bedside care, patterns of rigid and repetitive talk, and the containment and restraint of the person at the bedside, which were all ordinary and taken-for-granted routine aspects of bedside care for people living with dementia. However, these organisationally mandated ward practices, could, in turn, quickly exacerbate and intensify an individual's distress and reaction to care during their admission.

This suggests the 'looping effect', the way in which a classification can interact with the people being classified (Hacking 2007). Goffman identified this process of 'looping' within the total institution, describing it as 'an agency that creates a defensive response on the part of the inmate takes this very response as the target of its next attack' (Goffman [1961] 1991: 41). We identified these dynamic interactions locally within these wards. The institutional cultures of recognition viewed any response (resistance to timetabled care, and behaviour viewed as disruptive, inappropriate, or transgressive) to the organisation of wards and the routine bedside care within them, as both a feature of a dementia diagnosis and something requiring further management and control. However, these ward responses (tightening the timetables, rigid and repetitive talk, and containment, restriction, and restraint) generated further distress in the person, which led, in turn, to further tightening, containment, and so on. In addition, these practices also had powerful and negative impacts on ward staff, creating high levels of distress, anxiety and fear of 'falling behind' (which we discuss within Chapter 5). This produced a dynamic and powerful (and sometimes incredibly swift) interaction between the patient, the mandated organisation and delivery of care at the bedside, and the diagnostic category. These institutional cultures of care and their consequences supported and reinforced beliefs about both the classification of dementia and the recognition and application of this diagnosis and what constituted appropriate care for individuals.

This is, of course, associated with wider everyday beliefs and cultural understandings about ageing and the erosion of the person and the body. This also manifested within the wards, with staff typically interpreting losses in function or symptoms to people living with dementia as part of this underlying neurodegenerative condition (rather than a potential feature of their acute admitting condition). Family and carers consistently reported to us their frustrations that they believed medical and ward staff had limited expectations of the abilities of the person living with dementia during their admission. This resulted in assumptions around functionality and dependence; the inability to eat meals independently, assumed incontinence, and being unable to walk without 'falling', were all viewed as key features associated with their dementia diagnosis. This also extended to include mental capacity and the person's ability to make decisions, with mental capacity viewed as something that can be lost, and which, once lost, was a permanent deficit that related to all future decisions (Brindle and Holmes 2005, Poole et al. 2014).

Visibilities and invisibilities

Dementia as a visible public condition within these hospitals is at odds with dementia outside of it. In public life, people living with dementia are typically not visible, and experience powerful cultures of exclusion from everyday society whether living at home or within long-term care. This can be seen in the prevailing expectation of 'prescribed dis-engagement' following a diagnosis that Kate Swaffer (2014) describes. As she powerfully reminds us, 'Dementia is the only disease or condition and the only terminal illness that I know of where patients are told to go home and give up their pre-diagnosis lives, rather than to 'fight for their lives'' (2014: 3). Although a significant patient population within acute wards, they are also curiously absent from the popular imagination and cultural representation of the hospital. Wandering the wards of *Casualty*, *Holby City, House, Grey's Anatomy* and even docu-dramas such as *24 hours in A&E,* people living with dementia are notable by their absence. Perhaps the only accurate representation of the numbers of people living with dementia within hospital wards, and their visibility, is the black comedy *Getting On,* which, by no coincidence, was written by a former nurse.

As we have described, people living with dementia are a significant population in our hospitals. Although it was possible for us to visit an acute ward and for staff to report little to no admissions of people living with dementia, this was extremely uncommon, something staff would comment on to us as we entered these wards, welcoming a 'quiet' day or, more often, superstitiously hushing anybody who verbalised this for fear of 'tempting fate'. However, these assessments made at the start of a shift often did not reflect the population represented on the admission board and could also be subject to change and reassessment by these teams during the course of the shift. More often, the population of people admitted for an acute condition who also had a diagnosis of dementia within these wards, would number between 20% to 50% on any given day.

There was a disconnect, however, between the significance of people living with dementia within these wards and the level of recognition within these institutions at senior levels. Hospital managers and administrators would react with surprise when we, as researchers, proposed observing 'dementia care' in the acute areas of their hospitals. To them, dementia simply wasn't to be found there; surely we would have nothing to observe? Dementia was assumed to exist only within the confines of mental health, and specialist 'geriatric' care wards. This stood in stark contrast to the views and experiences of staff within these wards. Senior nurses in charge of the wards within these hospitals typically reported to us, often in exasperated tones that displayed how unsupported they felt by their institution, that as many as 50% of their in-patients also had dementia, whether diagnosed or suspected.

However, as we have described earlier, the assessment and recognition of people living with dementia within this setting is complex. Indeed, a hospital admission and the acute clinical admitting condition itself (and the interaction between them) are often key events in the initial recognition of symptoms associated with dementia and cognitive decline, and its assessment and diagnosis. Factors such as this confound and obscure the figures as potentially an over- or under-estimation of this population of people living with dementia within our hospitals. The local everyday practical recognition of dementia made by ward staff has powerful consequences, which will be discussed in detail throughout this book.

Yet, despite their prevalence, people living with dementia are habitually regarded amongst both senior hospital administrators and frontline staff within wards as the 'wrong' sort of patient, one who belongs elsewhere, who are 'a disruption to core business' (Gladman et al. 2011) and should not be taking up acute care services and beds designated for other more 'appropriate' patients. This has, of course, long been a prominent national discourse within the media, with older people and people living with dementia within our hospitals often referred to as 'bed blockers', who are taking up space needed by other, more deserving groups. These dehumanising and derogatory labels, frequently referred to within both the tabloid and broadsheet press at times of NHS crisis (although this term can also be found more widely within other European and Australian media reporting), are used to describe people whom we found desperately wanted to go home, but who were often confined within an acute ward by the slow-moving organisational and bureaucratic health and social care mechanisms, despite being classified as medically fit for discharge. Many others also developed an additional complication (such as a hospital acquired infection or delirium) associated with their admission, which further delayed their discharge.

Newspapers from across the political spectrum continue to give prominence and authority to this view of older people and people living with dementia in our hospitals. They appeared at regular intervals during our study across their front pages: 'Bed blockers cost the NHS £287 million', *The Independent* (Merrick 2015); 'NHS Crisis deepens as bed blocking costs NHS £6bn – Delays push hospitals to breaking point', *The Times* (Gibbons 2016); 'Scandalous waste of health cash – Bed blocking costs NHS £3 billion a year', *Daily Express* (O' Grady 2018); 'Hospital bed block shock – Social care chaos sparks new surge in elderly patients stuck on wards', *The Mirror* (Bagot 2018). We discussed this with Tony (pseudonym), a person living with dementia who has been a member of our consultation group throughout our ethnography:

TONY: We are people. And what I object to is and I think it's one which this government in particular, this one in particular has generated over the years, I've been described in the *Daily Mail* for those who want to read it as a tsunami, a disaster, an earthquake, a horror show. I've been blamed for the inability for the economic recovery because I'm a burden, all in very general terms and when you start saying those things over and over and over and over again

> that's how people... We are an asset, because you have a diagnosis doesn't stop you, doesn't prevent you from being an asset. Everybody's journey is different. Mine could be totally different tomorrow, I don't know but while I am where I am, I'm going to be who I am, and nobody is going to take that away from me, not without a fight anyway.
>
> (February 2019)

Of course, the world of these wards and the staff within them reflect these wider social understandings of both the purpose of our hospitals and who they should be caring for. Nursing students (pre-clinical placement) consistently reported to us that they expected to be caring for people of working age. These students were overwhelmingly surprised and shocked when we suggested that the key population when they enter these wards would be older people, and more specifically people living with dementia. We found that following their first hospital placement or rotation, they had quickly been acculturated by the setting, and when asked to describe who they were caring for, they typically sighed and complained about there being 'too many' people living with dementia and 'too much dementia' in these wards. The dominant cultures within these hospital wards viewed people living with dementia within them as a population who do not belong, should be cared for elsewhere, by other specialist teams within dedicated wards with dedicated resources. As we have discussed, however, this population need to receive both specialist care and treatment for their acute admitting condition. As we have found elsewhere, when older people with acute conditions and additional complex needs are transferred to wards dedicated to the care of older people, they can become further disadvantaged and excluded from the available treatment pathways and specialist medical care they need (Cramer et al. 2018).

These beliefs in the inappropriateness of this population to be cared for within acute hospital wards are deep-rooted and are not only a contemporary preoccupation. Roth and Eddy, in their classic ethnography 'Rehabilitation for the Unwanted' (1967), described their large public chronic-disease hospital in the USA as a 'repository for the unwanted'. They examined the institutional treatment of (predominantly older) people 'whose chief disability is that they are unwanted'(1967: 8), by other institutions and society more widely: the 'larger and larger numbers of disabled, poverty-stricken persons, who are no longer wanted by anyone and for whom a 'solution' must be found' (1967: 3). This has significant consequences, which we will explore in detail within this book. Typically, nurses expressed sympathy and concern for their patients, but the same obstacles were always raised, that staff did not have the time, did not have the training or resources, and that these wards did not have the staffing levels to care for people living with dementia. Too often this meant ward staff would discuss people living with dementia in their care with a shrug of the shoulders, reflecting this acknowledged discourse.

Staff continued to hold onto the belief and expectation that this population was a temporary phenomenon within their ward and 'should' be transferred (or, in the colloquial jargon of wards, 'moved upstairs' or 'sent downstream') to other more appropriate wards designated for 'the elderly' 'the geriatric' or to specialist 'dementia wards' that either do not exist for that purpose, nor have the number of beds that would be needed for this population if they did, within most hospitals. It also reflects the cultural primacy of dementia as a master status (Goffman 2009) overriding the recognition of an individual's acute admitting condition which requires specialist treatment and care.

In parallel, there has been a move towards establishing an array of new types of wards for older people, and with them appears new classifications, and admission criteria focussed on grading and organising patients by age, ability, and condition. These wards have labels that denote their role and patient population, such as COTE (care of the elderly), RAID (rapid assessment, interface and discharge), CI (cognitive impairment) and Frailty (older patients perceived to have an elevated risk of injury and decline). In addition, many acute wards, including the ones within our study, have a range of additional resources associated with being a 'dementia-friendly' ward (typically this meant appropriate signage and day rooms being refurbished to reflect *c.*1950s) and access to additional hospital-wide resources and interventions (specialist support teams), which we will discuss in more detail within Chapter 2. However, in the context of the rapid changes of leadership and staffing within these wards, we found that the specialist resources to support this patient group could quickly become unused, repurposed or locked away. Specialist teams or roles within these hospitals were typically only available during the shifts or rotation of this team, which, strikingly, often excluded weekends, evenings, and nights.

Cultures of care and systemic inequalities

Throughout this book we will explore the inequalities people living with dementia experience within these wards; however, the poor recognition and systemic under-treatment of pain amongst people living with dementia (Morrison and Siu 2000, Banicek 2010) illustrates the inequity in care that they are known to experience (Department of Health 2009: 62). Pain is poorly identified and undertreated in people living with dementia (Sampson et al. 2015). They receive poor end-of-life care, fewer palliative medications (Sampson et al. 2006), and less opioid medication (Morrison and Siu 2000) in comparison with other patients with the same admitting condition. People living with dementia may find it difficult to articulate their pain (Banicek 2010), or find that their articulation of pain is ignored or expressed in a way that staff do not understand, recognise, or prioritise. One study identified that people living with dementia receive only a third of the opioid medication provided to other patients who do not have a diagnosis of dementia (Morrison and Siu 2000), concluding that the majority of people living with dementia were in severe pain post-operatively (Morrison and Siu 2000; Sampson et al. 2015).

When we met June earlier in this chapter, she was able to articulate her pain, but not in the way the medical team required (she was unable to state where her pain fell on a ten-point scale). We revisit June following her transfer to the Trauma and Orthopaedic ward, following her total hip replacement. June is alone in a side room and as we sit with her at the bedside she tells us that she is in considerable post-operative pain. As the wider literature demonstrates, this is a common experience. What this literature does not capture, however, are the wider cultures of care, the ways in which care is organised and delivered at the bedside that impacts on these experiences and makes them so resistant to recognition, intervention and treatment. In observing June's care we can see the ways in which the organisational culture that prioritises the timetabled order of the medication round, places June's immediate needs for pain relief as 'a potential source of disruption' (Roth and Eddy 1967: 49) to the routine work of this ward.

> The next day I visit June, now in the ward, at 7.30 p.m., June has had a total hip replacement. Her hair is now combed neatly back and she is wearing a pale blush coloured nightie. I say hello and hold her hand and tell her I saw her when she arrived.
>
> She tells me, in a quiet voice, 'Oh father oh father oh father oh father I am in terrible pain, terrible pain, terrible pain.'
>
> I leave the cubicle and go to see the nurse in charge of her care and tell her that June is in pain before I go back to her. Again she repeats, 'Oh father oh father oh father oh father I am in terrible pain, terrible pain, terrible pain. Oh father oh father oh father oh father I am in terrible pain, terrible pain, terrible pain Oh father oh father oh father oh father I am in terrible pain, terrible pain, terrible pain.'
>
> I go to see the team responsible for her section again and tell them about June's pain. They are busy with the medication round and are seeing each patient in a set order (moving from each bedside to the next around the bay, visiting the single rooms last). After the main bay has been completed, the nurse comes and checks June's medication chart and brings back a syringe of diamorphine and empties it into June's mouth. June is now extremely distressed and fiddling and pulling at the tube attached to her nose (nasal cannula) used to deliver oxygen. The nurse puts this back in place and tightens the cord under June's chin to keep it securely in place before leaving. June asks for water, 'I am terrible thirsty', and I give her some water using a straw. I tell her that she has now had her painkillers and that I will stay with her until the pain goes.
>
> She repeats: 'The pain is going, the pain is going, the pain is going, the pain is going, the pain is going, the pain is going, the pain is going, the pain is going, the pain is going … you have lovely hair. Oh father oh father oh father oh father. Oh father oh father oh father oh father. Oh father oh father oh father oh father. Oh father oh father oh father oh father. Oh father oh father oh father oh father. The pain will go soon. It will go soon, but when, when, when, when? They have left me, the pain is in me. Somebody do something for me I AM IN TERRIBLE PAIN, TERRIBLE PAIN, HELP ME HELP ME HELP ME.'
>
> She eventually relaxes and closes her eyes. I leave feeling shaken and quite helpless.

June's experiences of urgency in conflict with the organisational priorities of the ward was repeated throughout her admission and extended to June's continence care. Her urgent and repeated cries for pain relief and help to visit the bathroom (she has a urinary catheter in situ), became part of the background soundscape of this ward. Her articulation of pain and being unable to recognise the catheter appeared to emphasise her dementia diagnosis to the ward team, with the repetition of her cries understood as a 'behavioural' feature of her dementia, rather than a need for urgent care, and she became one of the many people living with dementia within these wards viewed as an 'unreliable witnesses to their own experience' (Saukko 2008: 77).

> Two hours later, around 9 p.m., the lights are low and it has been quiet in the ward. I can hear June crying out from my position in the middle of the ward 'I AM IN TERRIBLE PAIN, TERRIBLE PAIN, HELP ME HELP ME HELP ME.'
>
> I go to check on her and when I enter the side room I realise she is screaming. I rush to the nurses' station to tell the healthcare assistant, and she tells the nurse that June needs more painkillers. However, they are busy with another patient and it is a while before they wheel the medication trolley into her room.

In June's case, staff appeared unable to prioritise, recognise (or believe) her urgently articulated needs. Within this book we will show that June's experiences were not an isolated incident, but indicative of wider cultures of care, which have powerful and detrimental somatic impacts on people living with dementia during an acute hospital admission. For people living with dementia difficulty in communicating a wide range of needs contributes to already high levels of anxiety and distress generated by these unfamiliar ward settings. This regularly led to people shutting down and retreating in on themselves, or becoming distressed and increasingly vocal in their requests for support (an individual often referred to within these wards as a 'shouter') from their bedside. The most common response was to resist some (or all) forms of care at the bedside. Importantly, these responses to care were typically recognised as symptoms to be managed and subdued. Resistance to care, for example, was always seen by staff as a core feature of dementia, something that staff would take pride in recognising and overcoming, but very rarely investigated the potential underlying causes.

Timetables, rules, and restraint

The consequences of these wider organisational cultures meant that staff held deep-seated expectations that all must fit within the 'rules' of these wards, conforming to the rigid task-based timetabled established routines of bedside care. As Roth and Eddy note, 'If a patient is new on the ward, he must be taught the customary behaviours and ordering of relationships' (1967: 49). Of course, that may be relatively unproblematic for patients without dementia or any form of cognitive or communication impairments, but for people living with dementia this was typically much harder. However, adjustments were rarely made to suit individual people living with dementia or to tailor the organisation and delivery of care to meet their needs as a wider patient group within these wards. Instead, we found distinct parallels in the patterns we observed with the classic work of Isabel Menzies Lyth, and her long-term engagement examining nursing within a UK general hospital in the 1950s and 1960s.

Although the contemporary population of people living with dementia requires increased flexibility and continuity in the delivery of their care at the bedside, the wards we spent time in typically responded to these increases in variation in individual patient needs and the fluctuating workloads that go with them in much the same way as observed by Menzies Lyth over half a century previously, by 'increased prescription and rigidity and by reiteration of the familiar. As far as one could gather, the greater the anxiety, the greater the need for such reassurance in rather compulsive repetition' (Menzies Lyth [1959] 1988: 63). William Caudill (1958) similarly notes these patterns within the small psychiatric hospital; the tightening of the timetables and routines in response to potential disruption or disturbance and we will examine this in more detail within Chapter 5.

When a person living with dementia was unable to comply with the tightly timetabled care at the bedside, ward staff would employ multiple interactional approaches that were all focussed on reinforcing the rules of these wards and we will explore this in more detail within Chapter 6. Ward staff employed a rigid and highly repetitive repertoire of language, tactics, and performative work, when carrying out bedside care. A reliance on stock phrases, simplified language, and slowly enunciated words delivered in a collective institutional timbre and the 'special tone of voice' (Goffman [1961] 1991: 19) of the 'total institution', but at the same time also used highly coded language all patients were expected to recognise, understand, and respond appropriately to, as we will show in the many examples presented throughout this book.

The organisation and delivery of task-based routinised bedside care, which Lyth (1959: 65) referred to as 'the task-list system', was always the key priority within these wards. This meant staff were also trapped within the fast-paced demands of the bureaucratic hospital systems. The need to meet the demands of the organisation overrode the immediate or urgent needs of any individual person, but in particular the complex needs of the person living with dementia. Despite the contemporary policy and nursing practice goal of delivering 'person-centred care', we routinely found wards driven by organisational timetables and targets that meant that this was impossible. Thus, although individual members of staff would acknowledge the patient reaction to (or counter to) the delivery of fast-paced routinised care, or their underlying concern or need in their talk at the bedside, they typically quickly oriented the person to the reality of where they were, what had happened to them, and, most importantly, what *must* happen to them at that moment. Although it was usual for staff to seek permission from patients for care to be carried out on their body, and staff gave the appearance of seeking permission, the expected pace of work meant that the delivery of care was typically already happening, with a tacit assumption of assent, with any further talk focussed on obtaining the correct response from the person to allow care, which was already being carried out, to continue.

When people living with dementia were unable to fulfil these requirements and expectations, individual staff and wards drew on a limited repertoire of talk to respond and contain them at the bedside in order to continue core ward routines and to stabilise the timetable. Staff typically presented instructions to be followed and obeyed, often emphasising the potential imminent danger of patient actions and these typically contained a powerful sense of urgency that often displayed staff's own underlying anxiety and fear of delays. Appeals to the necessity and expectations of the institution were commonly referred to, and these appeals emphasised that there was no choice for either the person or the ward team caring for them '*we have to change you*'. This talk was directed at reminding the patient of their place in the world and the status of ward staff, they must all fit the expectations and timetables of the institution. We will explore the 'privileges' of other patient groups in more detail within Chapters 5 and 7. These approaches created damaging cycles of anxiety for both patients and ward staff (Menzies Lyth [1959] 1988). This could lead to contagion and patterns of 'collective disturbances' (Stanton and Schwartz 1954, Coser 1962) where a 'mood sweeps in the general atmosphere... the majority of patients on a ward become upset at one time' (Coser 1962: 88), which has a long history as a phenomenon recognised within institutional life (Stanton and Schwartz 1954: 294) and we will explore this in more detail within Chapter 7.

Within all wards and across all shifts, we identified powerful cultures of containment, restriction, and restraint and we will discuss in more detail within Chapter 7. Although specific techniques had some variance between these wards, the overall strategy was always the completion of the timetables of care and to keep the person living with dementia within their bed or sitting at the bedside. Across all these sites, staff expressed high levels of concern and anxiety about people attempting to or leaving the bed or bedside, and this increased exponentially if they were walking in the bay, the wider ward and corridor, or close to the ward exit/entrance. Importantly, these approaches to patient care and their containment at the bedside was both a response to their diagnosis of dementia and perceived resistance to care; but were also frequently the trigger of further resistance, and associated with both patient and staff distress.

The work of bedside care

Importantly, these organisational expectations had powerful and detrimental impacts on ward staff. Staff were also trapped within the demands of the wider bureaucratic hospital systems, the local organisation cultures of care, and the fixed and tightly timetabled routines of the ward, which are associated with emotional burnout and exhaustion. It was not uncommon for staff to want to avoid assignment to bays or areas of these wards that admitted high numbers of people living with dementia, or for assignment to these areas to be rotated, or assigned to agency staff. We identified that ward staff typically did not feel supported to develop the skills or to deliver care at the pace and in the ways this patient group needed. A key ward response to high numbers of people living with dementia was to outsource their care and assign additional agency staff to shadow and contain people living with dementia at the bedside.

While there are many other groups entering and working within these wards (but who can also leave the ward), it is the domain of nurses and healthcare assistants, and it is these groups (who cannot leave) that we follow. Given the increasing delegation of 'hands-on' care in acute hospital wards to healthcare assistants, an important focus was this less privileged (Daykin and Clarke 2000) and marginalized group (Lloyd et al. 2011). The bedside delivery of care, the paid work carried out on the bodies of others (Wolkowitz 2006) and its wastes are habitually regarded as low status, bordering on the polluted (Twigg 2000). This is often gendered (Simpson et al. 2012) and invisible, skilled work that often appeared not to be valued by the wider organisation or by other hospital staff (Jervis 2001). We found that there was little recognition that the large number of tightly timetabled and repetitive care practices (organisationally mandated) at the bedside could have powerful consequences for all.

We also wanted to understand the ways in which staff made sense of their work. To identify the ways in which practices at the bedside took shape within and across shifts and became manifest, entrenched and understood as standard practice in the everyday care for people living with dementia. We identified the difficulties for ward staff in seeing the person, with the dementia diagnosis overshadowing and dominating responses and care delivery. Yet ward staff also experienced pervasive invisibility and powerlessness within these wards. The fixed organisational cultures and tightly timetabled routines of the ward, which are the most damaging for people living with dementia and their families, also had profound impacts on ward staff. Staff attention was driven by fulfilling the demands of the local organisation and routines of the ward, and there was a widespread and often-palpable underlying anxiety during shifts that their work was also under constant surveillance and scrutiny within the ward and also by the wider bureaucratic systems. We share with Menzies Lyth (1959) her preoccupation with anxiety and the ways in which the timetables, their rigidity and repetition caused, but also functioned to contain, anxiety within the hospital institution. Her 'attention was repeatedly drawn to the high level of tension, distress and anxiety among the nurses. We found it hard to understand how nurses could tolerate so much anxiety and, indeed, we found much evidence that they could not' (1959: 45).

We focus on the everyday cultures of bedside care, because this is where the routine, but vital, highly skilled patient care takes place. Where the work on the body, variously referred to as 'dirty work', 'elimination work', 'body work', or 'body labour' (Wolkowitz 2006), occurs. This is where the detailed interactions between ward staff and patients typically took place. By examining the ways in which the delivery of this care manifest in tasks, timetables, and routines, we were able to follow its cumulative impacts and consequences over time, on patients living with dementia and on ward staff.

Note

1 The dementias are a complex classificatory system with wide and diverse categories of disease and complex symptomology, in which the nosological boundaries are widely debated and in flux, which are examined in more detail in later chapters.

2 Ward life

Here we enter these contemporary hospital wards. We describe these institutions, from the built environment of these hospitals to the organisational structures that inform and regulate them, specifically the documentation, technology, and the staffing of these wards. We explore our processes of entering these wards, learning their 'rules' and the everyday institutional practices within them. We also describe the soundscapes we found within them, and the sensory experience of being within these wards. Through this, we will start to develop an understanding of these institutional cultures, the place of the patients within them and the ways in which this setting is particularly unsuited for people living with dementia.

> This hospital, just outside the busy centre of this large commuter town, is striking for its similarity to all the others we have already spent time in. There are no features that distinguish it, that recognisably tie it to the local area, or even to any particular era. It is made up of a jumble of assorted and often interconnecting buildings, some mid-century, others more recognisably contemporary and built in the last decade, in the limited utilitarian materials ranging from red brick to concrete. Across the campus there are also a number of small 'temporary' prefabricated buildings that are over a decade old. Between them all, any available space is designated for staff and visitor's cars. Across the grounds outpatients and visitors search for entrances and buildings, hesitating at the many signposts they follow pathways that loop around, under, and through, the many buildings on this campus.
>
> Approaching from the main car park the most prominent building is the Accident and Emergency department, perhaps the most familiar service provided by these acute hospitals, but also one that prohibits entry. Instead, to find the main entrance, patients and visitors must continue past the banks of ambulances, passing patients in pyjamas sitting outside in wheelchairs smoking. On this occasion one patient is smoking directly through the tracheotomy inserted in his windpipe. Come night-time these same hardy, barely dressed smokers will return, but their numbers increasing with that days admissions, and joined by others loitering at the hospital's edges (discarded silver cylinders of nitrous oxide, or 'laughing gas', indicating substance abuse littered the side alleys of at least one of these hospitals).

The main entrance seems untouched by modernity. It is not one of the apparently 'new' hospitals, whose similarly unplanned layouts are masked by glass façades containing brightly coloured sofas, high street food outlets, and murals reflecting the local area and its history. Instead, this hospital has the same design layout it has had for decades. Walls coated in aging magnolia and institutional green paint house a cramped and full waiting room. Those patients and visitors able to find seats sit on uncomfortable brown moulded plastic chairs, attached four to a row along a fixed metal frame. A café serves tea from an urn and instant coffee in polystyrene cups, along with an uninspiring range (cheese or ham) of pre-packaged sandwiches and tray-baked cakes. A set of stairs, elevators, and two corridors lead off from it, linoleum flooring leads to more green painted walls with brown plastic handrails, interrupted by brown wood-effect doors leading to toilets and signposted office and storage space.

While the décor is uninspiring there is little chance to take note of it, because the corridors are full of people moving in many directions, past patients lying on trollies awaiting tests and scans, or discarded beds (presumably faulty ones, given the nearby signs requesting that staff stop leaving faulty beds in the corridors). While signposted, these busy corridors quickly become labyrinthine. On my first day I am directed to turn right at the coffee shop, take a further two rights, a left, and then two more rights. A disorienting journey, but one which ultimately only took five minutes. At times, the intense busyness of the central corridors suddenly disappear and transition into long empty corridors lacking any natural light, where motion-sensitive lights have switched themselves off, creating a sense of unease, that you are not meant to be here, that this place is off-limits.

Past this, one reaches the ward. Being an older hospital building this ward looks like any other. A single long corridor dissects the ward, with double doors at either end, and another set permanently wedged open in the middle. The magnolia and green paint of the corridors continues inside, alongside pastel-coloured furniture, brown décor and decals, and cream-coloured metal beds. The ward is starkly and brightly lit, and feels very busy, not just with ward staff, but also with hospital staff passing through from and to other areas of the hospital. To the left side of the corridor are four bays, each containing six occupied patient beds (it is extremely rare to see an empty and unused bed waiting for an admission), from which patients and visitors watch those passing by. To the right is a long wall covered with an overwhelming volume of laminated A4 posters and signs, the most clear and prominent being those asking patients if they would recommend the ward to family or a friend.

Crossing the threshold for the first time I felt a trespasser, an intense moment of intruding where I did not belong; yet once within it, this ward felt deeply public. Against the unfamiliar backdrop of institutional colours, staff and visitors to the ward pass by each other, and patients sit waiting in full view of one another. It is difficult to describe how this ward simultaneously appeared one easily recognised as a traditional ward but also many novelties in the details, which was filled with so many people waiting, yet so full of energy of people moving at a fast pace, all at the same time. Around the central nurses' and clerk's stations gather numerous staff, all in different coloured scrubs, uniforms and tunics, complete with colour-coded piping, to denote their role and grade. However, for the patient, visitor, or researcher new to the ward, these colours mean little; there is no way of decoding and matching uniform to role, nor the responsibilities attached to each. It adds to an overwhelming feeling of being an outsider, and again the contradiction that a place so overwhelmingly ordinary and familiar, could at the same time be so uncomfortably alien.

(Site E, day 1)

Learning the 'rules' of the ward

The passage above describes the first 30 min at the fifth hospital in our ethnography, making our way to the wards, and attuning ourselves with their cultures and the wider institution of which they were a part. This was not only to be the fifth hospital, but the ninth and tenth wards in which we had worked, over a period covering almost twelve months. Still, amidst the familiarities of the neutral colours, the beiges and browns (or, in striking contrast, the new institutional colours of the new builds, equally anonymous bright whites against primary-coloured feature walls), and the layouts of bays and beds, where so much that was familiar and routine, each institution had expectations, features, characteristics, and the 'ways things are done around here' that were distinct, setting them apart. We still found the initial walk through this hospital disconcerting, confusing, and overwhelming and felt a powerful sense of not belonging, of breaching unspoken rules, as we walked through the double doors of the ward to introduce ourselves to the team.

Until one has got to know more about the 'rules' of each of these wards, there remains an uneasy sense of not belonging, a nagging doubt of requiring permission to open doors or enter areas, a hesitant sense of trespassing when walking onto each new ward, or the areas within it. Despite our familiarity with spending extended periods, weeks and months, within four other hospitals, we could not immediately get a fix on the codes that would tell us the rules and conventions of these wards. We could not tell the nurses from the healthcare assistants, the pharmacists from the therapists. We did not know who could be approached at the nurses' station, what the many signs on display meant, or what the unfamiliar names, abbreviations, and acronyms scribbled on whiteboards could mean. Furthermore, we found that even within the same hospital we were typically working within wards that each had their own distinct ways of working, their own rules and conventions.

The sense of disorientation and uncertainty on admission to these wards can be overwhelming, and, of course, all patients have 'to learn, and in some way conform to, the rules, restrictions, and freedoms of the hospital' (Stanton and Schwartz 1954: 170). We often observed patients living with dementia asking ward staff what they were allowed to do, if they were allowed to leave the bed or bedside, if they could visit the bathroom, if they had to pay for meals, snacks, and cups of tea, and if they could leave the hospital and return home. We will discuss the ways in which staff transmitted the 'rules' of these wards to people living with dementia in more detail within chapter 6.

This sense of dislocation is not limited to patients and visitors. One can observe agency staff, student nurses, and foundation year doctors demonstrating the same disconnection from their surroundings, not knowing who they can talk to, the conventions for addressing colleagues and patients, how to order tests and equipment, request services or consultations, where things belong, and the many other rules that coalesce to form the order of these wards. At the same time there exists a sense that the other staff, and even the other patients and visitors, must already know the conventions and expectations of the ward.

Entering the institution

NHS hospitals in the UK suffer from the quirks of their construction, built, extended, and re-modelled, outwards and upwards across decades. Red-brick buildings are linked by bare institutional corridors to mid-century brutalist towers, late-century prefabrications and onwards to the glass and steel frontages and atriums of contemporary extensions and new builds. The result of this expansion means that corridors do not always match, that going through one door often also means changing the floor number, and that corridors can lead to dead ends, sudden exits, fire doors, or prohibited areas.

Hospital corridors snake through buildings designated with arcane naming systems, with wards named after long-dead local dignitaries, landmarks, castles, colour codes, letters, or a mix of any and all of the above. Some sections are old, dimly lit, and claustrophobic, but can lead directly to bright open atriums, spaces modelled on shopping malls and Silicon Valley-inspired hang out spaces. Here the visitor (and some categories of patient) can help themselves to branded food, a coffee at Starbucks, or a sandwich and sushi from M&S Simply Food, to eat sitting on a comfy, primary-coloured sofa. The entrance façade and atrium, with their reception areas and shops, are typically the most modern section of these hospitals, typically adorned with a bronze dedication plaque to commemorate the official completion and opening ceremony found in all of these hospitals, '... opened by HER MAJESTY THE QUEEN ...', or a litany of increasingly minor royals and dignitaries. Move on through double doors to the next building and these signs of modernity are replaced by quaint throwbacks to older mid-20th-century hospital design, the 'Friends of the Hospital' café, staffed by volunteers, the charity bookshop (or shelves filled with donated books), the Chaplaincy (these always look circa 1970s), the modern juxtaposed with what was once modern. All of these lead to the elevators, where visitors stand, typically confused by the call system and signage, and eventually to the many wards that make up the institution.

Entering these wards

Upon entering each ward, of significance is 'the generally Spartan character of hospital life' observed by Stanton and Schwartz (1954: 54), and which is still apparent within these contemporary sites of care. Whether these acute wards were within an older mid-century brick building or a newly built glass and steel façade, they were still universal in their austere look and feel. While the age of the ward can be sensed through small details such as faux-wood panelling or the use of bright colour schemes, the overall legacy of the Nightingale ward is still apparent.

Many of these wards still resembled the traditional Nightingale ward layout, large open plan rooms containing anything from 6 to 22 beds. In total, each ward usually contained 28 to 30 beds. However, the majority of these wards are no longer completely open-plan. Instead they were typically divided into semi-public bays, each containing between four and six beds. On these bays the beds are organised into symmetrical rows positioned against opposing walls, arranged so that patients directly face the opposite bed. These bays often had some screening from the wider ward, but remained semi-public, visible from the main corridor, offering little privacy in practice. Each of these wards also had a smaller number of single occupancy rooms, typically reserved for the infectious (Clostridium difficile or 'C diff' is the most common hospital-acquired infection which can spread rapidly), those assessed as 'disruptive' to the ward or as being 'end of life' (although this was rarely if ever articulated).

On entering these wards, the first thing patients or visitors reach is not a welcoming reception, clerk, or nurses' station, but noticeboards, beds, and patients. Through the corridor, noticeboards covered with 'Thank You' cards from families, notices for awareness campaigns for sepsis, falls, and dementia, and notices that abuse of staff will not be tolerated. Charts documenting the number of falls, pressure ulcers, and under-staffed days that month are displayed alongside laminates stating visiting times, or that valuables and electronic devices are discouraged and brought in 'at your own risk'. The nurses' station is typically at the centre of the ward, so any newcomer entering it must first pass rows of noticeboards on one side and rows of patients, often in varying states of undress, on the other.

Regardless of the ward, each bed and bedside within it is of uniform design. Although some beds will be metal framed, and others plastic, they are all adjustable in height and positioning and all have side rails that are typically raised and left in place. The new versions are coated in smooth, cream plastic, and have a hint of late-century science fiction about their automated design, but their function, positioning and purpose remains unchanged from the earlier models. Above the bed will be a whiteboard (or magnetic board) bearing the patient's surname, first name, any urgent medical instructions, such as whether the patient is 'nil by mouth' or suffers from diabetes (and potentially also a symbol representing dementia) and their mobility needs (whether they need help or equipment to leave the bed or bedside). It may also name their medical team.

To one side will be a bedside chair, a large armchair with wooden armrests and cushioning coated in wipe-clean plastic in an institutional hue of blue or green. On the other side of the bed will be a bedside cabinet, often a bag of clothing or toiletries will rest immediately on top of this. This is often a tell-tale sign of a patient's age, functionality, and capacity. Younger, 'self-care' or 'self-caring' patients will have visible evidence of their own possessions with bags of clean day and night clothing alongside a display of toiletries, gadgets and gifts. Older patients, and particularly those who are living with dementia, will have only what they arrived in. Their possessions will have been placed out of reach within the bedside cabinet for 'safety' by staff and what they are wearing will belong to the institution, in the shape of hospital-issue nightwear (robes, slippers, grip-soled socks) and limited toiletries, such as a 'welcome pack' of toothbrush, mini toothpaste and disposable razor. A process akin to 'stripping' of older people, which is a far older institutional practice (which we will discuss in more detail in chapter 3) (Robb, 1967; Roth and Eddy 1967).

At the side of each bed will sit a mobile tray table, which can be moved on four casters from the bedside to within reach of the prone patient. The tray table is critical for patients living with dementia often with limited mobility or contained within their bed. The items placed on the mobile tray table will be the only ones they can reach and interact with from the bed or bedside. This is usually limited to a jug of water or orange squash, a beaker, perhaps a cup of tea or coffee or something more clinical, such as packets of cleaning wipes, disposable bowls, a bottle of antibacterial foam, and continence products such as urine 'bottles' and continence pads, left over from a previous interaction with the ward team and left ready for the next. Again, it is the younger patients, those assessed as 'self-care' or 'self-caring' who have 'privileges' (which we will discuss in more detail within chapter 7), can get up and move around freely, that have books, newspapers, magazines and electronic equipment (smartphones, tablets, laptops) on their mobile trolleys. The older patients, who are typically on the ward longer and have the least mobility while there, have the most spartan and impersonal bedsides.

Technology within these wards

Despite the representation of the modern hospital as a site of great technological advancements, there was typically little evidence of medical modernity within these wards, nor of its use or presence at the bedside. There was always a huge amount of electronic or digital technology visible, and during our time on these wards there new devices were often brought in (including hand-held recording devices, new types of mobile monitors and computers); however, novelty fades quickly within this setting. There was always an air of impending redundancy of the technologies entering these wards, and they too quickly acquired obsolescence even during our relatively short time within these wards. Paper and pen still predominated despite the presence of mobile computer stations, new systems and technologies, and the subsequent institutional obligations to receive training and utilise them, which accompanied their introduction, which were viewed with scepticism and weariness by ward staff used to working in certain ways.

Mobile machinery always lined the (typically narrow) corridors intersecting these wards; over time, however, it became apparent that much of this was broken or outmoded. The most visible technologies to be seen were the many mobile computer stations, and although there was much variability in their use, within many wards they were rarely, if ever used or switched on. Passwords were scribbled on Post-it notes and attached to monitors or written directly onto equipment with 'Sharpies', due to the rarity with which they were needed or in recognition of the large number of staff who may need to use it once. The red 'sepsis trolley' (to support the early recognition, diagnosis and treatment of sepsis) and the 'crash cart' (to be used for resuscitation and often covered with a blanket to protect sensibilities, a type of modesty cover) were ubiquitous in the corridors, untouched and often dusty through lack of use.

In contrast, the practical, everyday, always in use, mobile monitors, machines, and equipment essential to the delivery of bedside care, littered these wards. This includes the mobile observation monitors used to record blood pressure, heart rate, and oxygen saturation, and the machinery to transport patients and to support mobility, such as 'steadies', rotundas and hoists (there are very few wheelchairs used within the wards, these are primarily used by porters to transport people between wards and services within the hospital) and continence devices such as commodes.

However, equipment that was in constant use quickly looked worn and shabby. Much of this everyday essential equipment was broken and discarded in the corridor, typically left to gather dust in tired-looking and seldom used day rooms, or the nooks and alcoves of the corridors. Overall, there was typically a shortage of essential equipment, with the teams often having to search or ask colleagues from other teams in the ward, or neighbouring wards, and to borrow and barter for their use. Similarly, these wards would often experience shortages of other essential supplies, including fresh linen, towels, hospital-issue gowns and pyjamas. This could also extend to crucial technologies of care, including continence pads, disposable bowls and linings for bedpans, and commodes.

Even the most visible technology of the modern era, the mobile phone, was curiously absent from these wards. Staff are prohibited from looking at their phones during shifts, and older patients and people living with dementia are usually admitted without them. This makes these wards one of the few remaining public spaces where people are not frequently glancing at small screens, although the usage of the landline telephone, the seemingly archaic pager and the pneumatic tube delivery system still prevail. As a result, the sound of the unanswered landline telephone ringing at the nurse's station is an almost constant part of the soundscape of every ward.

Recording practices

Even when mobile computers and hand-held devices and screens were used by ward staff, the main administrative documentation practices visible within these wards remained the hand-written bedside records and medical notes. Mobile trolleys, filled to the point of groaning with huge amounts of paperwork, stand in corridors, stuffed with patient medical records, as well as the nursing Kardex, and the bedside folders containing hand-written patient records. Importantly, much of the key patient information for each shift was hand-written and added to the paper 'handover' document, a sheet (or bundle) of A4 printed off by or for each staff member at the start of each shift containing brief and basic tabulated information on all patients within these wards. Typically, this meant the most up-to-date information on a patient was tucked inside the pocket of an individual staff member.

Recording practices were a central activity for all, and although there seems to have been little technological change over the years, the volume of recording required appears to have risen greatly. Nurses' and healthcare assistants' conversations are littered with complaints about paperwork and the increasing amount of time taken up with recording bedside care and patient monitoring activities. Digital record-keeping is primarily the domain of the ward clerk, with their PC at the nurses' station typically the only one within each ward that seemed to be in common usage, running on outdated versions of Windows and Office software. While there was some variation across these sites, and although we did see digital recording practices entering some of these wards, paper records and recording predominated.

Organisation and staffing of these wards

The rhythm of ward life is characterised by patterns of apparent linear organisational structures of shifts, and timetables, influenced by the pace and priorities of different teams within and entering it (Zerubavel 1979), but also larger external forces. During our observations junior doctors went on strike, and a cold weather front led to a surge in 'black alerts', whereby hospitals no longer admitted patients, and where it was not uncommon in the areas observed to see patients receive treatment on trolleys in corridors due to a shortage of beds. At the start of our ethnography this pattern of increasing demand and shortage of beds was referred to as a seasonal 'winter crisis'; during later phases of our fieldwork, however, this developed into a recognition within these wards that this pressure on services was almost continuous and becoming an all year round experience.

During weekday shifts, the volume of people, the individual members of staff and 'teams' both based within, but also external to, and entering these wards, is striking. The medical teams walk side by side down corridors in the style of *The West Wing*. Staff from the housekeeping service mop and sweep floors in silence. Porters push huge beds that take up the whole of the available corridor space. The pharmacists, therapists, and phlebotomists, all walk briskly along the corridors, or stand reading folders or transcribe ever more notes into patient files. Ward staff rarely stand still and do so only to write notes or prepare and deliver medications. All work to their own remit, priorities, pace, and timetable of work, but at the same time they also appear to be 'going along with tolerable smoothness' (Caudill 1958: 28).

While the differentiation of these roles is signposted by uniforms, each a different bold colour, with minor decorative changes on lapels and epaulets differentiating grades and specialities, on first entering a hospital and the wards within it for the first time it is difficult to identify who is doing what, and whom you can speak to. At first glance, there appear to be two groups of staff within these wards: 'nurses' and 'doctors'. In reality, there is a loose hierarchy encompassing many roles, working under distinct demarcation, fragmentation, and specialisation. At first, the variety of roles might seem easy to spot. At one hospital the housekeeping team will wear purple scrubs, care assistants green. Nurses will wear scrubs in darkening shades of blue to demonstrate grade and rank (light blue for student and staff nurses through to navy blue for matrons, specialists, and nurse consultants), although a specialism or grade may be marked by a small stripe on a sleeve or a coloured detail that is unnoticeable to a visitor. Occupational therapists wear green trousers and white polo shirts, whilst physiotherapists are dressed all in green. Within the medical teams, the code is 'business casual': men all seem to wear blue Oxford shirts, sleeves rolled up and tan chinos, while women wear a variety of conservative office clothes. Beyond this, phlebotomists wear black tunics with red detailing, porters wear hospital-branded polo shirts, and agency staff dress all in white, while pharmacists wear mint green tunics. This is useful if you know what roles and remits these represent, yet each site will have their own unique system.

Beyond the recognition of roles and specialisms, comes knowing how these staff and specialisms work within these wards. The flow of information from patient to professionals and between ward teams and specialisms was frequently fractured. Patients and visitors presume that a request is made to a specific nurse or healthcare assistant (whom they likely assume are both nurses), this information will be passed on to the wider team. However, this is unlikely given the fragmentation of roles and the silos that exist within wards. Strangely when staff are approached (by patients, relatives, or other staff), a common response is often 'I don't work here' or 'That's not my patient'. Responsibility for patients within these wards is collective, which means it is also interchangeable and impersonal (Zerubavel 1979).

This fragmentation is visible in the clusters of coloured uniforms, coexisting on the ward but rarely meeting, moving in groups around one another, but rarely together. It can be seen in the contradictions: the therapy team that tells a patient to try walking around and stretching their legs, only for the healthcare assistants that follow them onto the bay to remind these patients that walking isn't safe and that they must remain in bed or sitting in their bedside chair. It can be heard in the patients who lament that they don't know who anybody is, or who all these people are.

Staffing within these wards

We identified wide variations in the staffing levels within and across these wards, and every member of staff we spoke asserted strongly that the current staffing levels within their ward were too low and often unsafe. While some of these wards were typically staffed by four nurses and four healthcare assistants, others would have two nurses and three healthcare assistants covering a ward of approximately thirty patients. Regardless of the staffing levels and structure within their ward, all nursing and care teams strongly believed they were short staffed, with the need for more staff viewed as the key solution to improving care quality within these wards. This was always part of the wider discourse within these sites, always central to discussions about caring for the specific needs of people living with dementia during an acute admission.

Each bay (and usually included two single-occupancy rooms) within these wards had a designated team, a nurse and healthcare assistant; however, depending on the levels of staffing, they may also be covering a wider area of the ward, which could extend to patients within other neighbouring bays and single rooms. This was particularly acute during staff breaks, when staff from one area of the ward must continue to care for that area while simultaneously covering another. This means that each small team may be responsible for caring for between six and ten, but sometimes as many as 15 high-dependency patients during a shift.

Some wards had consistently high levels of senior nursing staff present during shifts, whilst others relied on higher numbers of newly qualified nurses, healthcare assistants and students. Turnover of staff was also highly variable. Within some of these wards, turnover was so high that a staff member observed on one shift might never be seen again. In others, the majority of the team had worked within that ward for many years and, in some cases, decades. During our time on these wards we witnessed increasing staff turnover and reliance on agency workers, particularly those delivering 'enhanced care' at the bedside, or, as they were more commonly referred to within these wards, the 'one-to-one's'. It was usual to have at least one or two patients being 'specialled' with a designated 'one-to-one' agency healthcare assistant per shift, although in some of these wards it could extend to four patients per shift. Although this appeared to be a relatively new category of worker, this is a long-standing feature of ward management of patients who are viewed as demanding of staff time and can be traced to the experience of the mid-20th-century psychiatric hospital (Stanton and Schwartz 1954). This category of worker was increasingly used to respond to perceived staff shortages and to provide care to people living with dementia, and extended to patients with delirium or whom staff perceived as 'disruptive' to the wider work of the ward, conceptualising their behaviour as risks to be managed. Institutionally, people living with dementia were typically not classified as 'high-dependency' patients, and ward staff expressed their frustration that the organisationally mandated staffing levels did not recognise or reflect their often-complex and significant needs of this patient population within this setting. As such, the 'one-to-one' care system was relied upon as a means for staff to accommodate patients they felt did not belong in their ward, either due to the complexity of their admitting condition or their dementia diagnosis. This 'one-to-one' care rarely extended beyond sitting alongside a patient living with dementia, containing and restricting the patient at their bedside, enforcing the boredom and ennui. We will discuss the role of the 'one-to-one' carer, and the focus on containment, in more detail in chapter 7.

Soundscapes and senses

Each ward has a distinct institutional smell, a cocktail of disinfectant mixed with cooked food slowly congealing on plates left at the bedside. There is a general odour of bodies, mingled with something less pleasant, smells of infection, the whiff of acetone mixed with an underlying sweetness, the odour of concentrated urine, faeces, and diarrhoea coming in waves from behind curtains and through closed doors. Beyond this, there is the heat, which intensifies the atmosphere. The wards are kept at a steady overheated temperature (only new builds have air conditioning). Spending time on these wards is uncomfortable. Even during the winter months, the heat makes you sweat, and it makes your skin sticky. After spending more than an hour on them, the first thing you want to do upon leaving is to take a shower. In the summer months, it becomes unbearably oppressive for everyone.

These wards are always noisy. As described earlier, phones ring, personal alarms blare, monitors, machines and beds beep. The multiple and often-competing alert systems within these wards were unavoidable. Red lights flash on walls above bay doors and toilets, accompanied by beeps and alarms for staff. Landline phones at the nurses' station ring constantly, almost uninterrupted, throughout the day. Pagers beep and buzz. Monitoring machines beep and pulse to irregular rhythms. Personal bedside buzzers and chair alarms go off regularly and are re-set. IV machines call out when a patient rolls onto a tube or blocks a line. Bells ring as visitors arrive and buzz the clerk for admission. Patients scream, shout and sob, all imposed on to the background chatter of a busy workplace.

At the same time, as many as thirty staff members may be striding through these wards, standing around talking in groups, or in smaller groups of two working at a patient's bedside, combined with the additional background sights and sounds of visitors and patients talking at the bedside. Some patients might also have radios at the bedsides. This can lead to odd juxtapositions of a background soundtrack which jars with what is happening on the ward, such as the cardiac crash call observed as Fleetwood Mac's 'Go Your Own Way' played in the background, or the older patient using a walking frame to slowly and unsteadily walk along the corridor to Charli XCX's 'Boom Clap'. There was also some variation in terms of the availability of television within these wards. Wall-mounted screens were invariably tuned (by ward staff or to the limited channels mandated by the institution) to a free-view commercial station regardless of the suitability of the programme broadcast at that time. However, if they were tuned to daytime chat shows, the emotional content of confrontation, violence, and family issues could significantly add to the emotional charge of these environments.

There are also distinct patterns and rhythms of sound within the wards. At certain times during the shifts, despite the numbers of people working and living within them, wards can be quiet. Immediately after lunch, when clinical tasks and ward timetables are at a minimum, or at points in the night shift when there are no new arrivals, the timetabled work of the final medication rounds have been completed and patients are sleeping, the ward can become quiet. This can also be the case at the weekends, when the medical teams staff and allied health professionals do not work. This 'quiet' can bring a sense of calm to the otherwise fast-paced environment, although this word can never be uttered by staff, who fear that uttering it would be to tempt fate, for there was never a consistent pattern of when a ward would in fact be 'quiet' or how long this situation would last.

There were also distinct patterns within and across shifts within these wards, where 'collective disturbances' (Stanton and Schwartz 1954, Caudill 1958) would occur regularly and we will discuss this phenomenon in more detail later in Chapter 7. The most unsettling of these are the shouts and screams of patients that could cause distress for others, particularly those people living with dementia within these wards. During a night shift, for example, it was not unusual to hear those patients going through drug or alcohol withdrawal shouting out, demanding to be let out for a drink. In addition, people living with dementia or with delirium (hyperactive) may shout or scream for help and support throughout the day, just as patients left alone in side rooms call out to passing staff for attention. Each morning patients cry out 'No!" and 'Help!' from behind the curtains as the ward team attempt to complete personal care to meet the expectations of the wider timetable of the ward, and before the arrival of the breakfast trolley. Each evening visitors quietly cry in the day rooms and in the corridors just outside these wards, before patients cry as visitors leave without them. When a ward is quiet, it can take on an oddly calm quality; more often, however, the sounds of the ward can be overwhelming and deeply distressing.

For the staff, increased noise within these wards demonstrates the fast pace of their work and the continual demands the ward and the wider institution is making on them. As well as the timetabled work at the bedside, other patients need to be attended to as personal alarms ring, monitoring machines must be reset, patients needing help call for assistance from bathrooms. Increases in noise levels within these wards meant staff typically started to increase their pace, speeding up bedside care, and contracting the associated interactions with patents, dashing in and out of bays and along corridors, which, in turn, further amplified the noise.

> In the break room with the team we discuss the high-pitched alarms, they seem incredibly loud and oppressive to me. One of the healthcare assistant team remarks 'The buzzers haunt me, I hear them in my dreams!'
>
> Later that evening I find it hard to get the ringing sound out of my head.
>
> (Site 1 day 9)

For any patient, the noise on these wards can be disturbing. Shouting, screams, and the prolonged and often rhythmic screaming from one patient was a common feature of the soundscapes of these wards. A ward where a person (or multiple people) shout or scream is not a place where one can relax, where one expects to get better, but a place where one becomes fearful and afraid. This fear was often contagious, leading to other patients asking to go home, screaming for help, or sobbing in their beds. These sounds of human unhappiness, against the arrhythmic beeping of ward machinery and alarms, can make these acute wards a disorientating place to spend time. For this reason, these wards are seen as unpleasant places to work by staff across the wider hospital, with staff (particularly those working within the Medical Assessment Units) displaying their resilience in working in such an atmosphere as a badge of honour; however, they are still seen retreating to the staff room or even the sluice room to snatch a few minutes away from it.

> Amanda is in bed three of a six bed bay, of which five beds are occupied. She is lying flat on her bed, propped up by pillows with a nasal cannula under

> her nose. This is her second day on the ward and until five minutes ago she had a visitor with her, who has now left the ward. In response to this Amanda has begun to shout, almost pleading, to go home. She goes quiet when a nurse approaches her, but starts to shout again as soon as the nurse leaves her bedside, 'It's horrible, I want to go home', she cries, over and over again, like a mantra. This shouting prompts the lady in a bed on the opposite side of the bay to begins to shout as well: 'Take me home', 'it's shocking', alternating between one another, a call and response, occasionally swearing at the porter when he passes their bay. 'It's horrible, I want to go home' continues until Amanda instead shouts 'I want the toilet' instead, but by now nobody is listening. 'Horrible', she shouts.
>
> I speak to the nurse who tells me that she thinks all five ladies on this bay have dementia, although only three have a confirmed diagnosis. The nurse says that she expects the bay to be very noisy today. As the shouting continues, a lady on the next bay asks a nurse what all the shouting is about. The nurse explains to her that the lady has dementia and wants to see her daughter, and not to worry about it.
>
> (Site E day 14)

Acute wards are, by their nature, noisy, brightly lit, hectic and frightening places to be. This is felt almost universally by anyone who spends their days and nights within them. Towards the end of a shift, staff often appear physically exhausted and mentally drained. We too found that spending a shift simply observing the activity of these wards takes a toll, both physically and emotionally, watching a setting so simultaneously active and full of activity, yet also full of invisibilities and one where the person, the individual patient and member of staff, can become lost.

People living with dementia within these wards

For people living with dementia, admissions to the hospital are typically unscheduled. They arrive via ambulance and are admitted through the Accident and Emergency department, as we described in Chapter 1. Here they will receive their initial treatment, be triaged, and then transferred to the wards for further assessment, monitoring, and treatment. This will often involve admission to a unit (either critical or acute care, depending on the cause of the admission) for assessment and stabilisation before transfer to an acute ward where they will spend the majority of their admission. In total, people living with dementia are likely to spend time in two or three beds across two or three wards during an admission. This may include single-occupancy rooms or multi-occupancy bays.

They are admitted to these wards after 'falls', where their subsequent fractures are treated and cared for. They are admitted here with infections, low blood pressure, diabetes, strokes. They are admitted here with loosely defined conditions and taken-for-granted categories specific to older people assessed as having cognitive impairment, such as being 'confused'. They are admitted here for conditions that would not apply to a person without dementia, often sent from long-term community care with a diagnosis of 'general decline', 'odd behaviour' or 'loss of appetite'. There are many reasons why a person living with dementia will be admitted to these wards, which leads us to question why the cultures of care within these institutions appear unable to respond to the needs of this patient group.

People living with dementia are often admitted while they are unconscious or unaware of their surroundings. They will typically wake up, often alone, to find themselves lying in an unfamiliar bed, surrounded by other patients and staff, all strangers, in a totally foreign environment. Instead of wearing their own familiar clothes will find themselves dressed in hospital-issue gowns, typically gender-assigned in pastel hues of either pink or blue, propped up by pillows, with the bed raised to support their head and upper torso. The key organising principles ordering where patients were placed within a ward were always age, ability, and condition, thus (as we have set out previously in Chapter 1), people living with dementia are usually 'coralled' or 'cohorted' together within 'high-dependency' bays. This will mean they will look out to see two, three, five or more strangers lying in the beds opposite and around them, mirroring their own predicament, dressed in the same gowns, staring outwards with little to see or do.

Unless the patient wakes and shouts for help, which many people living with dementia will understandably do, it can be some time until the staff's rounds bring them to a person's bedside to introduce themselves to the patient and explain to them where they are and why. This is often accompanied by a long list of questions asking them to recall the circumstances of their admission, their home life, medical history, and medications. For many people living with dementia, this can be overwhelming, and they may respond with distress, with fear, or by withdrawing and attempting to hide away from this strange environment and the people within it.

People living with dementia as a group are also typically confined to their bed or bedside chair, and may remain for weeks, if not months at a time. Throughout this, however, they are left with nothing to do, nothing to look at, and nobody to talk to. In many ways, this resembles the 'massive inactivity' observed by Roth and Eddy (1967: 20) within the rehabilitation wards of the 1960s. Their observation of older patients limited to either lying in bed or sitting doing nothing and left 'often looking vacant and out of contact with the world' (1967: 20) is striking, because it reflects the contemporary experiences of people living with dementia and the cultures of care within these wards.

Even for those of us able to leave the ward at will, the ennui there is tangible. The progression of time is measurable in the timetables of bedside care, but between these fleeting fast-paced interactions, life in these wards is characterised for people living with dementia by an overwhelming nothingness, limited to simply sitting, sleeping and waiting. Within these wards waiting can quickly transform into anxiety and despair (Bandak and Janeja 2018). It is difficult to quantify this stultifying, overwhelming boredom. It is a boredom borne of the total lack of stimuli, the awareness only of time slowly passing, like waiting for a bus that never comes, and it creates the most startling contrast within each ward. Yes, the wards are hectic, busy, fast-paced, noisy, and public, yet at the same time they are overwhelmingly boring, monotonous, isolating, and lonely for people living with dementia.

The day for people living with dementia within these wards starts when the bright and often-dazzling overhead lights are switched on, usually at handover at 7 a.m or 8 a.m. They are roused from their sleep by staff in preparation for the day ahead. These wards typically operate a timetabled routine whereby all patients (there are no exceptions for people living with dementia within these wards) must be woken, washed, changed (this may include clothing and continence care), and, if possible, helped to get out of bed and to sit up in their bedside chair before breakfast is served. This routine is sometimes described as having clinical value, in keeping patients mobile (with a focus on rehabilitation) and avoiding pressure ulcers, yet at other times, the timetables of the auxilliary team (the arrival and leaving times of the breakfast trolley) and medical teams (getting the patients 'ready' in time for the morning rounds of the medical teams) clearly dictated this requirement. This fast-paced start to the day, marking the end of the night shift and the beginning of the day shift, starts a long day for people living with dementia, and for those caring for them. Although some of these wards dim the lights for a short period in the afternoon, the bright lights remain on until the ward timetable dictates it is night-time, anywhere between 8 and 10 p.m., when the lights are switched off and people living with dementia are expected to become quiet and go to sleep on cue.

As Roth and Eddy noted over 50 years ago, 'patients spend much of their time waiting' (1967: 201). To exacerbate this, these wards often have few windows, making it difficult for people living with dementia to judge the passage of time, something that can often only be traced by the timetabled routines of personal care, the arrival of meals, and medications throughout the day, or the regular nursing observations that occur every four hours. People living with dementia on wards that do have windows will often find themselves with drab curtains or pale blinds drawn all day, nothing to do, nothing to say, nothing to look out on. The ward begins to feel out of time, disconnected from the world outside. For people living with dementia, who are frequently asked by staff to recall the correct time and day of the week, this can be particularly disorientating, and contributes to their overall distress and uneasiness within the ward. However, these questions are also used clinically to assess their mental acuity and capacity, and could have significant personal consequences for their treatment.

Despite the close proximity and lack of stimuli, conversation with staff and between and across people living with dementia (and other patients) within these wards is infrequent and limited. In all our discussions with staff, they were all adamant that spending time with people living with dementia during their admission was key to care quality, and something many enjoyed, but they also explained that the demands of the ward timetables meant that 'no-one has the time' to do this. This is a long-standing concern for ward staff, as Stanton and Schwartz (1954) similarly describe. They observe that 'staff and articulate patients generally felt that 'sitting with patients' was the most therapeutic of the aide's activities' (1954: 163), but go on to describe that staff did not feel it was possible within the wards of the 1950s psychiatric hospital. We observed the same phenomena within these contemporary acute wards. Ward staff typically talked to patients only when they were delivering care to them at the bedside and rarely took part in, prompted, or encouraged talk across the beds to involve other patients in conversations. Instead, each bedside and the standard furniture immediately surrounding it was a curiously isolating island. Some patients would draw the privacy curtains, designed so that staff can protect a patient's dignity during work on the body, as partitions to avoid interacting with people living with dementia in neighbouring beds. This makes the ward a curious anomaly, it is inherently a social and public place, but at the same time it is one where little human interaction takes place. This may be why the boredom and isolation feels so tangible.

Ward life can be characterised as one of waiting and monotony, reflecting a well-recognised 'general state of boredom and tension' (Caudill 1958: 92). However, this is particularly problematic for people living with dementia. They are a patient group who may be waiting for tests and interventions for their admitting (and often multiple) condition; if they have been assessed as 'medically fit to leave', they may still be waiting for the complex processes of assessment for discharge to be completed. Many of these wards were locked, and locked specifically to keep people living with dementia within them, limiting the potential for what is typically characterised within these settings as patients 'wandering' or 'absconding'. However, this also meant that as a group they had no access to the wider hospital or the shops, cafés, and services within it. Even within the ward their personal belongings were typically out of reach and remain within their locker-style bedside cupboard, while the volunteer's trolleys that occasionally pass through these wards typically bypass them (as we will discuss in more detail in the next chapter). The typically extended admissions within these wards for people living with dementia could last for weeks or even months. This frequently meant a significant period of time with no opportunities to venture outside and experience fresh air or natural daylight.

Unlike other patient groups, few people living with dementia are admitted with their mobile phones (for many younger patients this is the first thing that a visitor will bring for them) so they cannot reach out to their family and friends outside. As we have discussed, some of these wards have televisions, with screens mounted on adjustable arms that can be pulled over individual bedsides (pay-per-view TV, where the PayPoint machines were always inaccessible for people living with dementia, being based outside the ward) or wall-mounted within each bay, typically with the sound muted and tuned to a digital channel, showing tired repeats of game shows, police procedurals, human interest reality programmes, and talk shows. As an alternative, there was the radio, which was usually tuned to a middle of the road radio station playing the blue-eyed soul hits of the 1980s.

The unsuitability of these wards for people living with dementia is widely acknowledged; in response, each ward always had a range of equipment specifically introduced to support people living with dementia during an admission, always referred to as the 'dementia-friendly resources'. There was some variation across these wards, but they typically included dedicated display screens with interactive games, 'reminiscence packs', picture books and drawing materials. However, these resources were rarely used; in the majority of wards they were neatly packed away, pristine or gathering dust, remaining in their boxes, with electronic equipment typically unused because remotes and batteries were missing. These were kept in the day rooms, which have mostly been refurbished to 'promote nostalgia' with a general feel and style that evokes the era of the Second World War, with false fireplaces, wall murals and retro casing for digital equipment, all typically circa 1940s and 1950s. The aim appears to be to bring to mind a conservative and rose-tinted notion of a halcyon era barely experienced by the contemporary older patient. These resting points or protected spaces were almost always unused, remaining empty for most of the day or re-appropriated as waiting rooms or bereavement suites for visitors. This appears to be a stable and recurring feature of ward life, echoing what Stanton and Schwartz observed many decades ago: 'The living room never functioned fully as intended' (Stanton and Schwartz 1954: 122).

For people living with dementia, these wards and the sights and sounds within them can be particularly distressing, disturbing, and frightening. People living with dementia were the group least able to recognise, or to learn, the 'rules' of these wards, and unable to fit smoothly within their institutional practices and organisational demands of the tightly timetabled and fast-paced bedside care. For many, the rational and reasonable response to the unfamiliar experiences of their admission was to try to leave it, to get out of bed and walk, to 'wander' away, to go home and return to the familiar. As Menzies Lyth concluded, 'normal behaviour in a hospital setting would be likely to include a good deal of expression of distress and protest, a *normal* reaction to an *abnormal* setting' (1959: 185).

3 Visibilities and invisibilities

As we have discussed, one key transformation within the contemporary hospital ward is the increasing number of patients on them who are living with dementia. Despite this, we found a reluctance at all levels across these institutions, across roles and disciplines, among both administrative and frontline staff, to accept that people living with dementia belonged, or could be found, within their acute wards. This disconnect with their patient intake was so embedded in the ways in which care was organised within these wards as to overlook the visible day-to-day nature of their work, and the nature of their typical admission. Within this chapter, we explore the complex ways in which people living with dementia were both seen and at the same time overlooked within these wards, at an organisational level and an individual bedside level. A key feature of an admission for a person living with dementia was the overriding sense they did not belong on these wards. As a group and as individuals they either were, or were made, invisible. This could also impact on the recognition of the patient as a person and on their immediate care needs.

It was unusual to see more than a small number of patients (usually just one person) of working age within these wards. On entering these wards, it was striking that the majority of patients were clearly older adults (as we have discussed earlier, within the context of these hospitals, the group classified as 'elderly' includes all patients over 65 years old) typically lying in rows, often unmoving, propped up within their bed or sitting in the bedside chair, wearing hospital-issue institutional clothing. As a group, increasing numbers of these older patients will also have dementia (we will explore the slippage between these categories within these wards in more detail within the next chapter). Their presence within these wards was also apparent in the soundscape of these wards. The repeated shouts from recognisably older and distressed voices, requesting 'HELP!' or to 'LET ME GO HOME!' were frequent, vocalising the most common and realistic fear for this patient population, that they would not go home. We observed nurses and healthcare assistants looking tense, dashing across corridors focused on containing these patients within their beds and at their bedsides. For someone unused to these wards, these sights and sounds can be unsettling and distressing; at first glance, the sounds and significance of this population of patients would appear hard to ignore.

These cries, however, frequently went unanswered. They were not typically ignored, since this would suggest staff had heard, acknowledged them, and felt they could answer them; rather, they had become part of the everyday background soundscape to what was considered to be the priorities and work of these wards. Similarly, the person living with dementia trying to leave their bedside may appear visible (and did appear so to us), but to staff, this was only at the point where they were recognised as having transformed into an immediate and pressing risk that must be managed. The moment they stood up the patient transformed, becoming visible, now a patient 'at risk' of 'falls', 'wandering' or 'absconding' to be returned and contained within the bed or bedside. This chapter will explore the ways in which the everyday cultures of these wards, the organisation of care work, and the delivery of routine bedside care within them, produced and maintained these invisibilities and examine their impacts on people living with dementia.

Seeing invisibilities

We found the profound invisibility of people living with dementia was striking. During one of our first mornings within these wards, the mobile shop (a large trolley full of snacks, drinks and daily papers) arrived. We watched as two volunteers steered it to the end of the ward, visiting each bay in turn, talking to and serving patients as they made their way around the bays and through the ward. However, of note was the level of anxiety their arrival provoked amongst a group of six older women within what ward staff informally call the 'female dementia bay'. Their loud and repeated calls for the trolley service went unrecognised by the ward team or by these volunteers. They did not stop. They simply carried on down the ward. Even with multiple patients calling out loudly and in chorus from their bay the volunteers just passed the 'dementia bay' by.

Amongst the women within this bay is Alice. Alice is 100 years old, has a diagnosis of dementia, and is recovering from surgery following a fracture. She is an extremely petite and elegant woman, with long silver hair in braids neatly pinned up and coiled around her head, wearing a quilted Paisley-patterned full-length day coat. A newspaper is an important part of her daily routine and she appeared ever vigilant and attuned to the rhythm of the ward and the risk that she may not get her daily paper. Her invisibility is repeatedly demonstrated to her (and to us) in the daily routine when the mobile shop visits the ward. Even when she left her bedside and the bay to stand in the corridor right in front of these volunteers and the trolley and call loudly, insistently, and with great clarity for a newspaper, she did not appear to be seen or acknowledged by them. The women within this 'dementia bay' were not viewed as patients with legitimate claims on or needs of their service, and they had to be extremely vocal if they were to make their needs known.

> Shortly after breakfast, the mobile shop arrives. The trolley the two volunteers are pushing is dazzling and brimming with sweets and crisps and full to overflowing. There is a pile of large family-sized 'grab packs' of crisps on top, then biscuits and drinks, the third layer is an array of types of mints and a range of daily newspapers and weekly magazines, with the bottom shelf

full of cans of fizzy drink. It also has a homemade contraption using moulded cardboard attached to one end of the trolley which forms a funnel filled with lots of different flavoured packets of crisps. It is a cornucopia of choice.

The trolley speeds very quickly through the ward and the two volunteers seem very focused on efficiency. As it rolls loudly past bay A, there is a gentle cry from the ladies within it. I am surprised and not expecting anyone to notice, but they are all clearly attuned to the rhythms and sounds of the ward. There is an outcry from everyone in the bay (referred to by staff as the female dementia bay). Alice calls after them 'paper … paper … paper ...'. She now looks very anxious and alarmed that they have continued to the end of the bay and missed her. The other ladies in the same bay, who have not moved or said a word all morning, now all join her and call out for a paper as well. However, they do not continue this for long. This appears to have taken quite a bit of energy and they lie back down, close their eyes and are still again. The staff passing by do not respond and I reassure Alice that the volunteers will be coming past again and are starting to serve patients at the far end of the ward and working their way back. The ward clerk looks across at me and adds 'Can you believe that she is 100!'.

When the trolley arrives in the bay, Alice is the most anxious to get her paper. She has set out all her change from her purse onto the bed. Once she has it, she immediately lays her paper out over the surface of her mobile trolley, puts her glasses on, and starts reading. The patients in two of the other beds also get papers, however, two other women who were calling out earlier miss out, one is hidden by the curtains drawn around her bedside and the team are helping her with personal care (washing and dressing) and the other is lying still in bed with her eyes closed, the volunteer team do not go up to check if she would like anything.

(Site A day 2)

The invisibility of people like Alice to hospital staff and volunteers was demonstrated repeatedly throughout our observations. Four days later, the paper trolley arrives as usual. Alice is walking using her frame, she has been back and forth to the bathroom all morning – the team tells me her diverticulitis has 'flared up'. She is walking very slowly and looks less steady than usual as she heads along the corridor. As before, she is dressed in her beautiful Paisley-patterned long dressing gown.

The mobile trolley is close behind Alice. The volunteers are about to overtake her at speed, but hesitate and pull up and trail closely behind. However, they start to overtake as soon as she moves to one side towards the bathroom, and she looks round and sees the trolley. She stops directly in front of them in the corridor and says very clearly and insistently: 'Paper! Paper! *Daily Mail*! *Daily Mail* please!' The volunteer pushing the trolley seems to be looking directly at her, but does not acknowledge her and appears to look right past her. The volunteer starts a long and involved conversation (over Alice's head) with her colleague on the paper round and a nurse who are both standing behind Alice. One volunteer is asking the other for change from a

> £20 note for one of the patients. Nobody acknowledges Alice. She is then ushered into the bathroom by a healthcare assistant and the volunteers and the trolley move on.
>
> After visiting all the other bays, the volunteer trolley leaves the ward without giving Alice her newspaper. When I realise that they are not coming back, I run after them, reaching them as they are heading into the ward opposite. When I say that Alice would like her regular paper, they look puzzled and tell me: 'I didn't see her, I wondered where she was!' I take a paper for her and they say they will come for the money later. I put the paper on her bed, the headline reads 'Busted Peer Coke Lord Sensation'.
>
> (Site A day 6)

The difficulty for these volunteers in seeing and recognising Alice as a person, or of acknowledging her needs and that of the other women living with dementia within this 'dementia bay', as legitimate, was repeated throughout our observations on this particular ward. They regularly missed out on the opportunities to buy newspapers and snacks from the trolley. This meant that they also missed out on opportunities for social contact and to connect with the outside world (via newspapers). As an observer, this was a daily pattern which became a highly stressful experience, particularly for patients like Alice. These experiences appeared to generate regular patterns of anxiety for Alice and the other women in the bay, waiting for the volunteers and their repeated efforts to be heard and seen by them each morning. This means that a service designed to support patients unable to leave these wards becomes instead a point within the day which emphasised the invisibility of some classes of patients. It also became stressful for us as, despite our earlier interventions, we would watch the same team of volunteers repeat this pattern which unfolded each morning and at some points we were required to intervene to ensure, as in the case of Alice and her newspaper, that patients' wider needs were met.

This pattern reflected the experiences of people living with dementia more widely; it was something we observed on many occasions across these wards. People living with dementia had to be extremely vocal and persistent if they were to make their needs visible to ward staff. However, even when they were trying to be heard and for their immediate needs recognised by ward staff, this (as we have seen with Alice) still did not mean their needs were recognised or prioritised within these wards. In contrast, patients who were able to clearly articulate their needs and were mobile and able to leave the bedside were recognised and served promptly by this service. We will explore in later chapters the myriad ways in which requests for support and urgent care made by people living with dementia (perhaps particularly for those who were less able to articulate precisely and quickly what they wanted) could be understood by staff as reflecting their dementia diagnosis rather than representing a legitimate need.

Speed and efficiency was clearly something these volunteers prided themselves on and this reflected the wider institutional cultures. However, their focus on providing an efficient service to all of the wards within these hospital buildings (a significant population and distance to cover each day) directed their attention to completing a specific task (the journey of the trolley), rather than the needs of the individual patients within them. Attention, as Zerubavel reminds us, 'functions like a spotlight. Whatever lies within its focus is well noticed, whereas what remains outside if effectively ignored' (2015: 4). This reflected the impacts of the wider institutional drivers of speed and efficiency that were felt powerfully by the people, patients, that appeared secondary to them. Within these wards, achieving efficiency was a key ward priority, reflected in the pace of work and the priority of timetabled, task-based bedside care. It was reflected in the pace of staff who rarely paused as they moved within it. It was typical for ward staff to appear visibly and audibly frustrated at the length of time a particular task at the bedside was taking, a projection of the anxiety that the ward timetables could be slipping, and the ever present fear of 'falling behind'.

We identified many ways in which the pace of work within these wards meant that people living with dementia (and older people) were no longer visible, and it was common practice for hospital staff across all roles and specialisms to cut and dart at speed past older people (some will also have dementia, but not all) who were walking slowly or using walking frames in the corridors as if they were obstacles hindering and delaying their work, or for silent and still patients to become inanimate objects indistinguishable from the bed that no one disturbed, but stride past, on to the next. Alice, for example, was described by this ward team as '*anxious*'; however, throughout our time within this ward she only ever appeared anxious and fretful about getting her daily newspaper. This precariousness informed Alice, and everyone within this ward, about which patients and what type of work was valued within these wards, further reinforcing the status of people living with dementia within the organisation and the work on these wards.

The invisible cascade of impacts

A hospital admission itself has significant adverse impacts on people living with dementia. The treatment or intervention for their acute admitting condition can, in turn, lead to an unintended sequence of multiple medical complications and a cascade of decline in the person, a process known as cascade iatrogenesis (Thornlow et al. 2009). In the case of an acute admission this cascade of events can result in further functional decline (Mukadam and Sampson 2011), dependency, institutionalisation, and potentially death (George et al. 2013). In people living with dementia (and older people), this can be triggered by what is a seemingly minor (and typically preventable) first event (Rothschild et al. 2000). These patterns of decline in people living with dementia were everyday and ordinary experiences within these wards, to the extent that they were typically viewed as a natural and inevitable, and, to some extent, viewed within these cultures as an unstoppable progression of complications and deterioration in this patient group. In the words of one consultant gerontologist put it during a morning round, her frustration and weariness clear to her team, this patient (a person living with dementia) 'now has delirium and sepsis, BUT his rash (his admitting condition) is doing better! Terribly ill! But the rash is *much* better and really good, until the delirium!'

However, there is evidence to suggest that for people living with dementia, this may not be a natural or inevitable decline that can solely be attributed to their dementia, but that the wider cultures of care during a hospital admission also contribute. There is evidence to suggest that these patterns of decline may be more closely associated with the organisational cultures that shape the delivery of care to this group. Of significance here is that the approaches to prevention of these patterns of decline emphasise the importance of ward staff having opportunities to see the patient and their needs, during routine monitoring and surveillance at the bedside (Thornlow et al. 2009).

These patterns of decline are associated with recognition and seeing. Nurses and healthcare assistants play a central role in this, and their delivery of highly skilled care at the bedside are key to the identification, recognition and prevention of potential adverse events and injuries in older people (Rothschild et al. 2006). However, we know that although adverse events are common for people living with dementia during an acute admission (Creditor 1993, Watkin et al. 2012), ward staff are typically not provided with the opportunities within the organisational restrictions of these wards to recognise, prevent, or treat, what are well-established and identifiable risk factors (Watkin et al. 2012). Within these wards we found little recognition of the risks associated with an admission for people living with dementia in their care, further demonstrating the systemic organisational failure to support ward staff in the recognition of the impacts of an admission, the hospital environment, and the delivery of bedside care, has on individual patients. It is a long-standing expectation, a shared understanding within these institutional and ward cultures that people living with dementia (and older patients) are the patient population who 'develops one complication after another' (Coser 1962: 122), transforming what may be preventable complications and decline in many of their patients, appear a natural and inevitable progression.

Observing these invisibilities could be legitimately distressing, and sometimes the most distressing invisibility within our observations occurred when a patient was doing their best to be seen and communicate their needs to ward staff. In the following example, Sophie, a woman in her early eighties, is lying on her bed in the middle of a large single-sex unit. Sophie is one of twelve patients being cared for by two nurses and a healthcare assistant within this part of the ward. We have discussed in the previous chapters how people living with dementia both belong and need to be admitted and treated within these wards, because they require specialist treatment for their acute admitting condition. However, there are also many people living with dementia who should not be in these wards and do not belong here. People living with dementia often arrive at these wards with no acute medical condition. Instead they are admitted as a 'social admission'; once treated and assessed as 'medically fit to leave', their discharge may be delayed due to either a risk-averse hospital culture, or the reluctance of some care homes to accept a patient's discharge, reflecting the disconnect between the domains of acute and social care.

The consultant gerontologist attached to this ward was unhappy because there was no medical reason for Sophie's admission. She was not being actively treated, having been admitted the previous week, and discharged once equipment had been installed in her home to support her independence, with a 'package of care' in place. (A 'package of care' (or 'package') is hospital parlance for a risk-assessed programme of care visits, specialist equipment and support to enable safe home living). Sophie's readmission was deemed necessary because her equipment had been installed in the upstairs of the house, which she cannot access, an administrative error, rather than a medical issue. During Sophie's readmission her husband tells the team that he no longer feels able to care for her at home, meaning an entirely new discharge pathway and care plan is required.

At the time of observation, Sophie had already been admitted to an acute assessment unit, with no pressing acute need, for 48 hours. It had taken until the second day of her admission for a team from social services to come to her bedside and assess her needs. They concluded that her case was too complex for them to assess there and then, and extended her admission for an additional 24 hours. The impacts of this admission itself, an entirely bureaucratic creation, cause Sophie to become acutely 'agitated' and distressed. In turn, her increasingly vocal distress as she sought attention from the ward team appeared to amplify both the invisibility of her needs and her invisibility as a person, setting her apart from other patients. She appears to be on an island on her own, 'cut adrift' (Coser 1962: 39) from the wider ward.

> Just before 8 a.m. Sophie begins to angrily shout for some water. The nurse in charge is behind the curtain with another patient, and shouts from across the bay that she can have some with her breakfast. 'Bloody ridiculous', the patient replies. After a few minutes pass, Sophie begins to shout 'Can I have some breakfast then please?' The breakfast trays are visible in the middle of the ward, the nurse does go and start serving breakfast, but rather than responding to or immediately serving Sophie, who continues to shout for food, the nurse instead begins the routine of serving each bed in numerical order, including patients that are still sleeping. Sophie occasionally shouts 'RIDICULOUS'. The nurse in charge continues to serve breakfast trays, one at a time, until she reaches the neighbouring patient to Sophie. The nurse is interrupted by a man in office attire, whose name tag gives his role as Operations Manager. He tells the nurse in charge that she needs to stop what she is doing and leave the ward immediately to help him with another patient. The nurse initially refuses but he insists. The nurse in charge then leaves the ward, pausing the breakfast round right before Sophie, who has still not been served. Sophie observes the nurse leaving, and continues shouting for water and breakfast with increasing stress: 'Are you all deaf or something?' The nurse neither looks back nor responds. She leaves the ward, following behind the Operations Manager.
>
> 15 minutes later, Sophie is still shouting for breakfast 'I've changed my mind, I don't want any breakfast, I just want some water'. A member of the housekeeping team finally responds to her, the first to do so 'You are not hungry anymore?', to which she replied 'I've passed it, I don't want it, it's too late'. 'It's only ten past eight.' 'It's passed.' Sophie continues to shout for water, and for a wash. This eventually turns to more general shouting and 30 minutes later Sophie is still shouting, about getting her clothes from her bedside cabinet: 'Who's got the key to my door ... Who's got the key to my

> cupboard … Who's got the key to my cupboard… Who's got the key to my cupboard … COME ON!... KEY TO MY CUPBOARD'. Nobody responds to her. 'Have you lost it?', she asks, quieter, before falling silent. The hot drinks trolley arrives in the bay. A minute later, Sophie loudly begins to ask about the cupboard again 'CAN I HAVE THE KEYS TO MY CUPBOARD, VICTORIA, COME HERE, SOMEONE'S GOT THE KEYS TO MY CUPBOARD, THEY WON'T GIVE IT TO ME, COME ON, THIEF, OI THIEF'. The Consultant, sitting taking notes at the nurses' station, says 'Oh bless her' to a nurse. After a few minutes, the patient stops and says 'It's OK, I've found it' and goes quiet again, although nobody has responded to her or tried to reassure her. Sophie continues to talk to herself after this, but she is inaudible and much quieter than previously, then announces 'I'll have a wash next'.

Sophie's frustration in her attempts to obtain the attention from the ward team does not fit with the conventions of ward conduct, but is recognised and accepted by ward staff as a behaviour to be expected from people living with dementia during an admission. Within these wards such actions are described as a 'challenging' behaviour, rather than an expression of a legitimate care need or grievance. This extends beyond the order in which food is served (but this alone is enough to legitimately cause great distress and could easily be addressed), to include her urgent care needs, which have direct impacts on her dignity and her well-being. These interpretations of Sophie's behaviour mean her pressing continence care needs are then also ignored:

> At 9:35 Sophie continues talking, but is no longer shouting and what she is saying is largely drowned out by the wider noise of the ward. None of the nursing staff respond to what she is saying, but eventually a member of the housekeeping team goes over to her as part of her rounds. Sophie can then audibly be heard asking about 'pads' and 'water'. The housekeeping member of staff thinks she is referring to the tray table, where Sophie has knocked her beaker over, but as she begins to clean this up Sophie peels back her bed sheets to show she has wet herself. The housekeeping member of staff understands and goes across the bay to tell the healthcare assistant and then comes back to the bedside. While she is away, Sophie complains about being left in such a state. Sophie won't allow the housekeeping staff to put the sheet back over her while she is wet, so is lying flat on the bed, exposed to the bay, on wet bedsheets. Housekeeping prioritises mopping up the spilt water from the tray table and the floor, causing Sophie to shout at her, asking why she isn't helping her. The housekeeping staff has to explain that she cannot, that she is not allowed to. Sophie turns to look down the bay and shouts loudly 'All I want is a (continence) pad, put it in there. Will you go and get me another, love?' The healthcare assistant standing at the end of her bed now says 'OK', but instead of doing so immediately, takes a form from the bottom of Sophie's bed. The healthcare assistant takes this to the nurses' station opposite her and starts to fill it

> in, in direct view of Sophie. While the healthcare assistant is doing this the nurse in charge sees her doing paperwork and interrupts. The nurse asks the healthcare assistant for assistance with another patient. When they turn and start to walk away from the nurses' station Sophie shouts, 'Thank you, thank you very much'. When she realises that the assistant has started going to help another patient Sophie gets upset and shouts loudly 'Aren't you going to change my towel? She had it in her hand!' She sounds incredulous. While the nurse in charge and the healthcare assistant are at the other end of the bay, Sophie continues to ask anyone that passes for help. A male nurse from another ward walks past her bed and Sophie shouts to him 'You could do it, couldn't you?'. He, with no knowledge of the context of the patient's needs, smiles at her and responds 'I can do it', and then carries on walking, his passing platitude unbefitting to the situation Sophie finds herself in. Sophie is now really angry and distressed, shouting that she is 'going to tell your bosses' and 'If you just give me it, I can do it!'

This situation continues to escalate through the morning. The more Sophie shouts out and tries to draw attention to her pressing needs, the more staff (there are many nearby) fail to recognise her, or view her calls as legitimate. It is well established that not responding to patients' cries or calls for help 'is a means of establishing authority with the patient' (Coser 1962: 77) through which the patient is 'taught the customary behaviours and ordering of relationships' (Roth and Eddy 1967: 49). Even when staff stand at her bedside they seem to block her out. In response, Sophie becomes increasingly frustrated, and her shouting demonstrates that this invisibility is clearly and powerfully felt.

> At 12:25 Sophie shouts across to the nursing station, asking why there is a bottle of cream on her tray table (a white squeezy bottle). She gets no response from the staff, who are gathered around the nursing station, opposite her bed, mere feet away. She gets no acknowledgement. Sophie then asks for cream on her food, prompting a nurse from the specialist frailty team, who had been on other side of ward, to come over and say to her 'That's not cream, it's soap' and take the bottle away. Sophie erupts in rage at this, pointing at the nursing station accusatorily: 'You gave me soap? Why would you do that?' She carries on, accusing them of trying to trick her into eating soap. By 12:28, this has escalated and she is banging on the tray table with her cutlery and shouting very loudly 'GIVE ME MY SOAP', occasionally quietening down to mutter about suing people, before raising her voice again, demanding to see the head of department and shouting at any individual member of staff who happens to walk past her. This continues, and the staff essentially blank her. It is not just that they do not respond, but that they effectively do not seem to hear her, despite her shouting from just a few metres away. Sophie appears to recognise this and starts to create even more noise, hitting the base of her knife on the tray table (a hard, loud rhythmic noise), but no one on the bay or at the nurses' station so much as flinches at this. By 12:42, she is furiously banging on her tray, shouting about soap and cream 'Come

on! I WANT THAT BOTTLE OF SOAP'., She is looking at and addressing three doctors who are standing at the station just a few feet from her bed, again with their backs to her and responding in no way to her shouts, as if she was not there and was not making a tremendous noise. 'Better not take it away, I'll find it, put in on the table, just there', she says, still rattling her cutlery on the tray. To staff within this ward it is if she is not there. The crash alarm goes off on the other side of the ward and all staff run over. It turns out it is a false alarm and they begin to drift back. By now Sophie is shouting: 'WHY ARE YOU IGNORING ME, DON'T SPEAK TO HIM, HE'S ON THEIR SIDE, IT'S THE PRINCIPLE OF THE THING'.

(Site C day 2)

The invisibility of a patient's needs was not always this pronounced: importantly, however, over five hours of observation of this patient's experiences, we identified a pattern identifiable across all of these wards and sites: the processes of escalation. The more invisible this patient feels, and indeed has become, the more this transforms into frustration and often-incandescent rage. Sophie expresses many valid, important, and fundamental care needs, for food, drink, and continence care, that she cannot obtain herself (she cannot leave the bed), but she also asks continually to be listened to and to be seen, for social interaction. However, in the context of a ward full of staff from many teams and specialisms, all with their own patient lists and priorities, and urgent calls (the Crash Team and the resuscitation of a patient) she becomes part of the wider soundscape of the ward, a normal feature of the setting, a noise to be expected, rather than a person in distress.

Sophie's experiences powerfully demonstrate the ways in which an admission can quickly have significant negative impacts on an individual patient and the ways in which the organisation and delivery of care within these wards meant that staff were often unable to recognise the needs of their patients, or indeed the impacts of the wards on the individual person in their care.

Cultures of not belonging

The difficulties ward staff had in recognising, or being aware of, the significant risks of adverse events and poor outcomes for people living with dementia in their care, can be associated with specialism hegemony. We found that acute staff within these wards often viewed dementia as a condition that was outside of their remit, not part of their specialism, but belonging to the care and specialism of other professionals or other wards within the hospital.

In the UK, dementia falls between clinical domains. As a condition it is traditionally viewed as belonging within the remit and specialist expertise of mental health practitioners (this typically includes the remit for staff training and the funding, planning, and commissioning of clinical services), and thus has not been viewed as an essential expertise or a significant patient population associated with acute clinical specialisms. However, the treatment of acute conditions such as pneumonia, infections (particularly urinary tract infections), and fractures (Sampson et al. 2009, Pinkert and Holle 2012) typically do not occur in isolation, and must take into account the potential impacts of an additional (or potential) dementia diagnosis. This extends to the recognition and treatment of a wide range of other co-morbidities (for example, people living with dementia are also likely to have conditions such as diabetes or hypertension). While there is an increasing emphasis within the wider literature on the importance of responding to the complexity of patients within the acute setting presenting with multimorbidities (two or more long-term conditions) (Bunn et al. 2015; Voss et al. 2017) this is yet to be reflected within these wards.

As Rose Laub Coser found in her classic study of a USA community hospital of the late 1950s and early 1960s "the elderly person' 'doesn't belong here' (Coser 1962: 123). This reflected the cultures within these wards still, sixty years later. The contemporary clinical and nursing literature has identified how these long-standing hospital cultures view the acute setting itself as an inappropriate place for older people (Tadd et al. 2011), who should instead be transferred to other services (Moyle et al. 2008). Despite the widespread rehearsal of this conventional taken-for-granted belief, these studies found little reflection amongst staff of where the most appropriate place for this group would be, and suggests an underlying ageism within these services (Tadd et al. 2011). We found that within these wards, these cultures were particularly directed towards people living with dementia. Staff typically pitied patients living with dementia, had low expectations for their prognosis and recovery, and, during breaks in their shifts, nurses and healthcare assistants across these wards reflect these beliefs, that they 'don't belong' within the setting, nor was it 'dementia friendly'; instead it was 'frightening' and resembled a 'war zone'. Importantly, this was always expressed as a taken-for-granted understanding that these wards were inappropriate for people living with dementia. There was, however, never any evidence of a discussion about how these wards, or the staffing practices within them, could be adapted to respond to and meet the needs of this patient population.

> I am in the small office which also serves as the break room with a sink, fridge and kettle as quite a few of the team have their break. I note that there are lots of patients over 100 years and we discuss the patients with dementia. They tell me:
>
> 'They say we are dementia friendly but they all should be …'
>
> 'They don't belong here …'
>
> 'It's a sad illness, cruel, looking at him ….'
>
> 'They get disoriented, it's frightening for us, for them it's probably more like a war zone!'
>
> 'We have the 'This Is Me' document, you need to get that filled in as soon as possible – it is useful and memory books to use with patients when you sit down with them. It tells you who they were and once you know that you can ask about the past, their job, the war …'
>
> (Site A Break Room)

As we have described within Chapter 1, when we initially entered these wards to discuss our study with staff, they often responded that if we wanted to study 'dementia care', we were in the wrong ward, and they would typically direct us to the one small 30-bed 'Care of the Elderly' ward within that hospital (the hospitals in our research typically had over 500 patient beds). Often the ward to which they referred, be it real or imagined, would be spoken of with horror, as akin to 'Bedlam' as both a scene of confusion and disorder, but also as an asylum, a place for the mentally ill. Porters, curious about our research, would often stop to ask why we weren't observing these other wards. They would pass on anecdotes about how unpleasant they were when they last transferred a patient to them, as in the example below, during an uneventful night shift.

> It is nearing midnight and the ward is quiet. The porters keep telling me I should be on the fifth floor if I want to see 'challenging behaviour' from patients. One porter, a man in his late fifties who seems to know everybody at the hospital, tells me that the fifth floor is where patients such as the patient I had been observing the previous night get taken. The previous evening this man had been shouting loudly throughout the night due to a catheter in situ. Throughout the night he would repeatedly be reminded by staff about the catheter but quickly forget, and in response constantly shouted about his pressing need to go to the toilet. The porter tells me that last night on the fifth floor there was, one bay of six men which had five 'shouters'. The porter added that he felt sorry for the other man, who was just trying to sleep.
>
> (Site A day 10)

Visibility and stripping practices

Importantly, as with those reduced to and viewed as 'shouters' above, key markers of personal identity of people living with dementia (and for other older patients) were routinely stripped away within these wards. The practices of 'stripping' older patients (of their personal possessions) (Robb 1967) is a long-standing one, which has consequences. The 'process of stripping the patient of moral and social identity' (Roth and Eddy 1967: 79) further emphasised the ways in which the needs of people living with dementia as individuals were narrowly interpreted by staff. The practice of allocating institutional attire impacts upon the perception of the patient by others but also by the self. It further demonstrated to the person their place within these wards.

People living with dementia typically had few (if any) personal clothes on their body or possessions visible at their bedside. On entry to these wards, they were given and dressed in hospital-issue gowns or pyjamas, with their other possessions placed out of sight within the bedside lockers (which were often locked or inaccessible). This ritual aspect of the admission process within these wards also represents a key feature of the total institution: 'On admission to a total institution, however, the individual is likely to be stripped of his usual appearance and of the equipment and services by which he maintains it, thus suffering a personal defacement. Clothing, combs, needle and thread, cosmetics, towels, soap, shaving sets, bathing facilities – all these may be taken away or denied him, although some may be kept in inaccessible storage' (Goffman [1961] 1991: 29).

Institutional clothing within hospital wards affects both the male and female body, but particularly the presentation of the ageing body, and has a powerful role in reinforcing the invisibility of people living with dementia (and older people). Across these wards, while there was some variation in the cultures of patient clothing and dress, it was standard practice for people living with dementia (and this extended to all older patients) to be dressed in hospital-issue institutional gowns with ties at the back that exposed the body (and thus often display any continence products, i.e. continence 'pads', typically a full body wrap-around nappy, that the person may be wearing) or pyjamas. Within these wards, they were typically only available in pastel hues of blue, pink, green, or peach, with some also stamped with the name of the NHS institution, sometimes with the logo in miniature forming patterns across the cloth, paired with hospital-supplied socks (usually bright red, although there was some small variation) with non-slip grip soles, all distinctly marking both the clothing and the person as 'belonging' to the institution (Goffman [1961] 1991: 28).

These institutional clothes were stored and taken to the bedside with the other linen during the routines of personal care. In the intensity and pace of the morning timetabled rounds of changing bedsheets and personal care, it was usual for people living with dementia (and older people) to be dressed (they often had little say in this) in a generic hospital gown or pyjamas. Within some of these wards this allocation was gendered, with the women all dressed in pastel pink gowns, and men in pastel blue pyjamas. Although the sizing varied considerably, a 'one size fits all' approach to storing these in bulk within linen cupboards with little to indicate sizing, meant they often hampered independence, people living with dementia often had difficulty walking while wearing long pyjama bottoms or needed to have their trouser hems rolled up to prevent tripping (this could, of course, also lead to staff seeing this as an additional risk and discouraging them from leaving the bedside).

This ill-fitting clothing was often felt powerfully by people living with dementia (and older people) and influenced not only their physical comfort, but also their sense of appropriateness and decorum, often causing longer-term underlying discomfort and distress, even though they may be unable to express this verbally. Kontos has shown how people living with dementia may retain a powerful awareness at a bodily level of the demands of etiquette (Kontos 2004, 2005, Kontos and Naglie 2007). Here Richard is wearing an institutional pyjama top, which was far too large for him. It had no collar and a very low cut 'V' at the neck; throughout the day he continued to try to pull it together to cover his chest. It was clearly making him feel uncomfortable, exposed, and vulnerable:

> The trolley is placed in front of Richard, but the plastic cloche is still in place over his lunch. He fiddles with his top, it is a very low top with a particularly low V neck because it is extremely large for him, he clearly seems uncomfortable with such a low top. Richard cannot open the plastic cloche and instead tucks into his pudding first. The healthcare assistant comes over 'Well that's OK, eat your pudding first'. Richard scrapes the pudding bowl clean and again he fiddles with his low top, the V across his

> chest is too low cut for him. As he eats he uses one hand to hold it closed, covering his body.
>
> (Site C day 5)

We observed that some patients within these wards appeared to be much more 'visible' to staff than others. It was often apparent how the wearing of personal clothing could make a patient and their needs more readily visible to others as a person. This may be especially so given the contrast in appearance clothing may produce in this particular setting. On occasion, this may be remarked upon by staff, and the resulting attention received favourably by the person.

> A member of the bay team returned to a patient (living with dementia) and found her freshly dressed in a white tee shirt, navy slacks and black velvet slippers and exclaimed aloud and appreciatively, 'Wow, look at you!' The patient looked pleased as she sat and combed her hair.
>
> (Site 3 day 1)

Such a simple act of recognition as someone with a socially approved appearance takes on a special significance in the context of these wards, particularly for patients living with dementia whose personhood may be overlooked in various ways. This question of visibility may also be particularly important since people living with dementia are likely to be less able to make their needs and presence known. The work of Twigg and Buse in particular has drawn attention to the role that clothing can have on preserving the visibility, identity, and dignity, of people living with dementia whilst both constraining and enabling aspects of care (Twigg 2010, Twigg and Buse 2013, Buse and Twigg 2015).

Some people and classes of patients were supported in wearing their own clothes, particularly if they had an extended admission, were classified as 'medically fit to leave', and were waiting for discharge arrangements to be made. There is a long tradition within hospitals of wearing personal clothing viewed by staff as an indicator of progress and rehabilitation (Roth and Eddy 1967). Of course, the more cognitively aware patients could more readily organise or request their own clothing, and would thus not have the need for embodied recognition that people living with dementia may have.

Not being dressed in familiar clothes was often profoundly felt by people living with dementia. Some people could see the humour and absurdity in their dress. For example, one woman living with dementia described the institutional feel of the hospital issue blue tracksuit she was wearing as 'I look like Olympians or Wentworth prison in this outfit! The latter I expect...' [Site C day 1]. For many, though, this was extremely distressing and emphasised to them the unfamiliar setting and their stripping away within it. They had no control or agency over the clothes that they were dressed in, nor where their own clothes were stored, which could be very frightening. Yet, as we see here, these concerns and anxieties were rarely understood or recognised as valid. Returning to the work of Kontos (2004, 2005), Twigg (2010) and Buse (2015), an important body of literature has also shown how people living with dementia strongly retain a felt, bodily appreciation for the importance of personal appearance. The comfort and sensuous feel of familiar clothing may remain, even after cognitive capacities may be lost. More strongly still, Kontos (2004, 2005), drawing on the work of Merleau-Ponty and of Bourdieu, has argued convincingly that this attention to clothing and personal appearance is an important aspect of the maintenance of a bodily sense of self, which is also socially mediated, in part via such attention to appearance.

Our observations support this work. Here, Catherine (who is living with dementia, assessed as 'medically fit to leave', but unable to return home and live independently and is waiting to be assigned a place in a long-term community setting) expresses her overwhelming feelings of exposure within this ward. The team have dressed her in a hospital gown (which is very exposing, because it is open at the back) and rationalise with her that this is because she has no clean clothes (her large network of friends have been regularly visiting and supplying fresh clothes). Her distress is immediate, and she is very tearful and anxious; this gown has very quickly emphasised her loss. The loss of independence, her inability to leave, raises valid concerns for her future: '*Will I get out of here?*' This is also something she felt materially and bodily. Wearing an institutional gown rather than her usual clothes, particularly not wearing a bra or trousers, emphasised powerfully to her both her exposure and vulnerability.

> I arrive at the ward and go over to say hello to Catherine and she says to me 'I still love you'; she is very teary and upset. The agency one-to-one carer assigned to spend the shift with Catherine is with her and tells me that she has just helped her to have a shower and because she doesn't have any fresh clothes she is now in a hospital gown. Catherine is sitting in a pink hospital gown with her lilac cardigan on top and it is clear she doesn't feel right without her clothes on 'I want my trousers, where is my bra? I've got no bra on'. She is very teary and upset.
>
> AGENCY ONE-TO-ONE CARER: 'Your bra is dirty do you want to wear that?'
>
> CATHERINE: 'No I want a clean one. Where are my trousers? I want them. I've lost them.'
>
> The agency one-to-one carer explains that her clothes are dirty 'Do you want your dirty ones?'
>
> CATHERINE: 'No I want my clean ones'. She is very teary and distraught.
>
> The cleaner arrives and starts to sweep around her and as he does this he says hello to her. She is holding on to her cardigan and drawing it around her and is very teary as she explains that she has lost her clothes. He listens and is sympathetic.
>
> CATHERINE: 'I am all confused, I have lost my clothes, I am all confused. How am I going to go to the shops with no clothes on!' She is crying and becoming increasingly upset and she gets up and goes to her bedside cabinet and starts to look through all the bags stored there. She goes back to the chair and the agency one-to-one carer sits opposite her. She is very distressed and tells us 'I have lost all my clothes, I can't get dressed to go to the shops. I am all confused, I don't know where I am. Why am I here? Why do I have to be here?'

AGENCY ONE-TO-ONE CARER: 'You broke your hip and it is now mending'
CATHERINE: 'Will I get out of here?'
The agency one-to-one carer leans over and holds her hand 'Yes'.
(Site 5 day 5)

The significant distress Catherine experienced over her absent clothes might be simply attributed (as it was by the ward team) to 'confusion', and this then may solidify staff perceptions of her condition. However, we need to consider whether rather than her condition (her diagnosis of dementia) causing distress about her clothing, the direction of causation may be the reverse: the absence of clothing contributing to her distress and disorientation, indeed Catherine recognises that her loss of clothing is causing her confusion at this situation. Others have argued that even people with limited verbal capacity and limited cognitive comprehension will have a direct appreciation of the grounding familiarity of wearing their own clothes, which give a bodily felt notion of comfort and familiarity (Buse and Twigg 2014, 2015). Familiar clothing may then be an essential prop to anchor the person within a recognisable social and meaningful space. To simply see clothing from a task-oriented point of view, as fulfilling a simply mechanical function, and that all clothing, whether personal or institutional, have the same value and role, might be to interpret the desire to wear familiar clothing as an 'optional extra'. However, for those patients most at risk of disorientation, it can be a valuable necessity.

The power of institutional clothing and dress in identifying and signalling to ward staff that a person was living with dementia could be most profoundly observed in the patients that proved an exception to this rule. The patient contained within the bed with the raised side bars, dressed in institutional gowns or pyjamas, hospital-issue socks, wearing continence pads, clearly signalled to staff that this was a person who had dementia. The impacts of this casual labelling and signposting of patients could be observed when a person within these wards did not fit within or meet these expected visible signifiers and expectations of this classification. Across these wards, staff would share their 'identity anecdotes' (Goffman [1961] 1991: 104) of patients living with dementia mistaken as a member of another group (visitor) and allowed or helped to leave and to 'wander' or 'abscond'.

One example of this was a woman, Janice, who had been admitted to an assessment unit. Janice was in her late 70s and had been admitted with a pre-existing diagnosis of vascular dementia. Her medical records suggested to the team that her dementia was in its advanced stages; however, her behaviour and functionality belied this. Within the ward she was extremely agile, coordinated and independent. Janice was admitted with an infection, which had been successfully treated; however, she then remained for an additional week because of the protracted organisational pace of obtaining a place in appropriate community care for her. Janice was clearly disorientated by the setting and she reasonably rationalised that she was in a hotel or on a cruise, rather than in a hospital, and was constant in this understanding throughout her admission. This reality sometimes made her extremely distressed, particularly when Janice was worried about who was looking after her house and, more pressingly, her dogs. Over the course of her admission it was never made clear if she still had dogs, or if this was a memory of previous pets. Nor was it made clear who may be looking after them in either case, despite occasional visits from her sisters. This fear over the welfare of her house and dogs meant she wanted (and tried) to leave the ward and return home, or as it was typically referred to by this team, try to 'wander' or 'abscond'. Unlike many other patients living with dementia, Janice was frequently able to leave the ward, leading to the urgent and repeated mobilisation of the hospital security team to find her before she left the building. Janice was able to leave the ward in part because each morning she insisted on having a shower, before spending an hour at her bedside, using the only mirror on the bay, over a small sink in the corner of the room, to style her hair immaculately, to apply her make-up, to change over the contents of her handbag and to dress in smart and expensive looking clothes.

The exceptionalism of her presentation became apparent in many ways. Firstly, each morning when I asked the ward staff to identify which patients within the unit had a diagnosis of dementia, they would look at the handover notes or the semi-public admissions board and tell me her bed number (as we have noted, it was very common and usual practice across the wards for patients to be referred to by bed numbers), before looking over at her and conveying their uncertainty by performing a double take or suggesting there had been a mix up or that patients may have moved (we will explore this phenomena in more detail in the next chapter). The simple act of being dressed and wearing make-up made her look much younger and more alert than the other patients within her bay, including those without dementia. Secondly, when this patient left her bedside or the bay, only the small number of staff (from a far larger population of teams and specialisms within the unit) assigned specifically to her care during that shift would interrupt her journey. She was typically able to navigate the large ward, and staff regularly held the security doors open for her, helping her to leave the ward and wishing her well. Her clothes and presentation masked the assumed signs and signifiers of dementia needed for its recognition by the ward team.

Prior work has also shown how older people, and in particular people living with dementia, may be thought to be beyond concern for appearance, yet this does not accurately reflect the importance of appearance for this group. Indeed, along with the work of others such as Kontos (2013) this shows that, if anything, visual appearance is especially important for people living with dementia.

Technologies to promote visibility and attention

Importantly, the invisibility of people living with dementia has been increasingly recognised by these wider institutions and one key response has been the implementation of an array of small, visible, and potentially temporary signs and symbols placed at the bedsides within hospitals across the UK to 'alert busy staff' that the patient they are caring for is also a person living with dementia. This represents an expansion of institutional approaches to make certain groups of people, or their needs, visible. For example, the use of red trays for delivering meals were introduced into wards as a 'visible indicator of vulnerable patients who needed help and support from all staff' (Bradley and Rees 2003), while The Butterfly

Scheme (using the image of a butterfly to represent 'dementia') was designed explicitly to inform the large number of staff arriving at the patient's bedside of their dementia diagnosis: 'In hospital, dozens of staff can pass through a patient's life each day and in order to deliver appropriate care, they need to know that a patient has dementia or memory impairment and how to support them.'[1]

All of these wards used some form of signage and symbols attached to the patient's bedside and displayed on the semi-public admission boards to indicate a patient who was also living with dementia. Here, a 'blue flower' (to represent dementia) and the 'red tray' (to represent the person requires support at mealtimes) symbols were both used within this bay. On the wall behind each bed, there were small pinboards (in other wards this is typically laminated wipe or magnetic board) and these symbols were placed with other signage indicating information about the person that all staff attending the bedside must know, such as 'Nil by Mouth', and descriptions of the person's mobility, or their personal preferences:

> On the board above bed 18 is a laminated forget-me-not blue flower symbol, which indicates he has a diagnosis of dementia. Additional notes written on the board says 'Best Stedy', indicating that the person's mobility is judged by the physiotherapy team as requiring equipment to transfer from the bed, and 'tea, milk, 2 sugars' indicating his hot drink preferences to the housekeeping team. He is sitting in the bedside chair in green hospital pyjamas. The trolley is in front of him and he slowly organises his box of biscuits and takes two out of the box and places them carefully on a plate.
>
> (Site C day 4)

There was, however, some variation in this signage, and their use and interpretation by staff within these wards. These signs must be understood in the context of the large amount of signage, laminate posters and notices that proliferated within the wards, indicating rules, regulations, targets, campaigns, and preferred practices. As in this case, during a discussion with the ward team, they recognised that they were all using this signage differently, which prompted one of the nurses to attach a blue flower sign (representing dementia) prominently above the bedside of one of her patients:

> The dementia awareness 'This Is Me' form and blue flower scheme are clearly signposted on a noticeboard attached to the wall between bays A and B (although dementia patients are typically cohorted on to bay C and bay D). The board consists of pictures of blue flowers and six very text-heavy laminated A4 notices. There are no blue flowers or 'This is Me' folders on any of the bays. The doctors and nurses at the station discuss that they are aware of the blue flower scheme but accept that it has not been implemented. The nurse from B bay decides that one man in her bay, Martin, should have a blue flower. He is an older gentleman who has only just been brought on to the bay from A&E. He is sat up on his bed, wearing hospital pyjamas, and seems to be in a good mood. He is alert, and happily chatting to the patient in the beds opposite him, asking questions about where he is. The other gentleman

> respond to him, one reassuring him, 'You shouldn't be here long' as another patient walks over to join the conversation. While they do this the nurse takes a blue flower sticker and attaches it to the board above the bed. Back in the corridor, at the station opposite the bay, one of the doctors in the medical team is worried that these flower stickers will be left up for a non-dementia patient admitted later, recounting how often the patient name is not changed after a transfer. The nurse says she will always do it on her bay from now on and will bring this up at the next ward meeting. She wants the whole ward to do this from now on.
>
> (Site A day 1)

As in the example above, this concern is legitimate and, within all these wards, we observed that the use of these symbols was not consistent, and quickly forgotten. We found that this array of symbols to represent 'dementia' within these wards, in corridors, on boards at the nurses' station, above beds, all helped to further reinforce the invisibilities of this population within the wards. We identified that signage and people often moved independently of each other and it was not unusual within these wards for a person living with dementia to be moved to another location or discharged, yet the laminated sign and label representing 'dementia', to remain, becoming detached from them, and instead attached to the next person. This not only risks misunderstandings within the ward, with patients inadvertently receiving inappropriate care or erroneous understandings of the needs of that person, but also risks the erosion of the visibility of the sign itself. If staff know the signs are often inaccurate, they cease to provide visibility, and instead contribute to the invisibility of dementia within these wards. There is also questions on what these technologies of visibilities achieve. After having the blue sticker put above his bed, Martin, from the extract above, began to attempt to go to the toilet, but could not get there as his hospital pyjamas kept falling down, embarrassing him. He would pull them back up and sit back down, unseen by staff. However, despite several clear and frequent requests to staff to go to the toilet, and the sign above his bed to show staff his needs, Martin is told instead he must stay sitting down as he is being monitored by machines. Thirty minutes later Martin wets himself.

Discussion: Visibilities and invisibilities

There were many individuals, classes of occupations, practices, and types of work, which appeared to be invisible and unrecognised within these wards. Within any organisation there are always groups whose everyday work or very presence is not recognised formally and is often unnoticed and invisible (Star 1999), and in these hospital wards we found that this included healthcare assistants, nurses, auxiliary staff, and also family carers. Auxilliary staff including housekeeping staff, catering assistants, and cleaners, could be invisible to nurses and healthcare assistants, who, in turn, were typically invisible and unrecognised by the medical and surgical teams entering the wards. Agency nurses and healthcare staff, a critical group in the care of people living with dementia (providing one-to-one care) in many of these wards, could be invisible to just about everyone and became just as invisible as the patient they were ostensibly caring for. This was in many ways a sign of them successfully fulfilling their mandate (to keep the person from interrupting timetabled care and to contain the person at the bedside) within that shift.

Within the confines of these wards, looking beyond the magnolia paint, the pastel pyjamas and gowns, the primary-coloured scrubs and the walls of laminated signage, there is a constant tension between what is visible and invisible. The organisation of these wards requires individuals to be invisible, to become a patient, a body in a bed, for the ward team to deliver care as it is institutionally mandated. However, a person and their individual needs must also be recognised to obtain appropriate care.

These processes of invisibility, generated from the restricted ideals of who belongs, who is recognised as having dementia, and the patterns of everyday delivery of care at the bedside for this group, leads to a loss of recognition of their needs as individuals. This could have significant impacts on care; as recognition of the patient as a 'person' declines, so too do their opportunities for recognition of care needs, rehabilitation, and the perceived suitable options for discharge. We identified powerful and consistent patterns where people living with dementia would be excluded from everyday social contact at the bedside, with the potential for the reduced recognition of their needs within these wards, as we have seen in the examples of Alice and Sophie above.

As we have described, although people living with dementia (and older people more generally) were not able to opt out of medically mandated routine bedside care (such as the medication round), they routinely appeared invisible to the wider social world of these wards. They missed out on the opportunity to buy a daily paper or snack from the mobile shop, or to borrow a book from the mobile library. We observed them being bypassed completely during the many ward routines that are socially important points of interaction, such as the opportunity for cups of tea and coffee, but also those services entering the wards that were specifically aimed at stimulating and supporting patients such as a visit to their bedside from the therapy dog or the chaplain. In practice, as with the mobile shop above, these opportunities were only ever available to the alert, awake, and cognitively aware patients who could make their needs known and articulated in customary and accepted ways. This invisibility and challenges in seeing people living with dementia during the everyday organisation and delivery of care at the bedside has consequences and produces vulnerabilities (Thornlow et al. 2009).

Note

1 The Butterfly Scheme, UK. http://butterflyscheme.org.uk/ site accessed 5/06/2018

4 Recognition and attribution of dementia at the bedside

Introduction

Here we explore the ways in which dementia was recognised and assigned to older patients within these wards. We found that it underwent a series of transformations that both produced and reproduced it as a public, taken-for-granted, and everyday diagnosis. It became a category all could recognise and see at the bedside and attribute to (or, in some cases, remove from) older patients within these wards. Within this chapter, we explore the consequences for patients and for the wards themselves.

There is a reification within the biomedical literature of dementia as having a range of diagnostic features, assessed via a series of cognitive and clinical tests, to be adjudicated, assembled, and recognised in the person by clinical specialists. Of course, this does not mean it is a stable category, and there is considerable complexity and variation within the recognition of the wide range of conditions and clinical features within this diagnostic category, with repeated and ongoing attempts at standardisation. Yet we found that within these wards, dementia became an everyday unremarkable category attributed and applied to large numbers of older patients, while simultaneously recognised via a remarkably contracted and restricted range of presenting features. During patient assessment and reviews at the bedside, staff focussed on the identification and assessment of cognitive features associated with the condition, primarily on memory loss in the abstract that was assessed and understood linguistically through recall. More widely within these wards, it was recognised in the older person's behaviour, focused on judgements of their interactions with ward staff; non-verbal or embodied communication, was not recognised as such, but understood and viewed as forms of behaviour (resistance to timetabled care, and behaviour viewed as disruptive, inappropriate, or transgressive) to be managed and limited in the person.

These understandings were the same regardless of each person's clinical history, presenting condition, or, indeed, whether they had a formal diagnosis of dementia within their medical records. There was also little differentiation or acknowledgement of the different types of dementia or the range of impacts they could have on the person, with a broad category of 'dementia' typically referred to and applied. As a result, a patient diagnosed (elsewhere) with Lewy Bodies would be expected to demonstrate the same features as a patient diagnosed with early stage Alzheimer's disease, within a general label of 'dementia' typically applied to patients within these wards. With the key impacts of the condition understood as generalised cognitive loss in the older patient. These understandings informed wider beliefs and expectations of the person as having significantly diminished cognitive capacity (with the person assumed to have 'lost' their ability to make rational decisions about their care), characterised by high physical dependency, and correspondingly low functionality and mobility regardless of stage or type of dementia. This, in turn, has consequences. This broad category of patient was associated with corresponding understandings of appropriate care (which we will discuss in the following chapters) within these wards.

These understandings of dementia and its impacts on the person was an everyday working model large numbers of non-specialist staff applied to older patients in the course of delivering everyday assessments and care at each bedside. As we have noted within Chapter 1, an unremarkable and consistent feature of bedside work was the repeated querying and testing of memory. These informal tests cast doubt on the mental acuity of all older people within these wards, with an expectation that a deficit would be identified. Dementia was an unremarkable and taken-for-granted category applied to larger social clusters or 'cohorted' groups of older patients within these wards. This was an accepted diagnostic category, a routine and everyday practice of naming and claiming applied to large numbers of older people. During our observations, we found that, at some point, the behaviour of any older patient who, for example, became distressed, or demanded to go home, could be attributed by ward staff as indicating 'dementia'. Rosenhan famously noted the 'the stickiness of psychodiagnostic labels' (1973: 252), and the ways this informs perceptions of the person that have a life of their own, shaping understandings of the person that endure throughout an admission and following discharge. However, what was particularly notable within these wards was that it was also a surprisingly fluid category and it was possible to see dementia identified in a person within a shift, but also apparently 'cured', with the diagnosis disappearing at 7 p.m. when the shift was handed over to the next team who made their own assessments of these patients. It was a diagnosis that could be queried if the person appeared to be high functioning, or showed increasing capacity or mobility during an admission, or at the point observations took place. Across these wards, it was common for different members of staff or the teams working within them to have diverse understandings of an individual's diagnostic status.

Importantly, within these wards, dementia was a condition all could name and claim to see. The transformation of the 'dementia patient' to include large numbers of older people within these wards reflects the status of dementia here, as a public condition, with a correspondingly narrow and limited range of taken-for-granted classificatory features. The world of these wards reflects wider cultural understandings of dementia and ageing. It reflects within the wards an assumed helplessness. This manifests in assumptions of the ability of the older person to care for themselves, in the degenerative and terminal nature of this condition, and the perception that decline was 'natural' for this condition and an inevitability during an admission and thus potentially a limited role for ward staff to intervene in its lifecourse. By examining the practical and mundane everyday ways in which dementia was attributed and responded to at the bedside, this allows us to explore the consequences for patients and the wards themselves.

Nosographic categories

Conditions, diseases, and syndromes are constructed out of the symptoms they contain. However, clinical entities such as Alzheimer's disease or Lewy Body Dementia are ideal types. The classic textbook classifications for conditions such as these are typically established on the basis of relatively simplistic clinical criteria and descriptions. As we have argued elsewhere (Featherstone and Atkinson 2012), there are multiple, often-discontinuous, forms of medical understanding that coexist, are intertwined, and that have complex and powerful impacts on how conditions are understood and recognised in practice.

Within this book we focus on an examination of 'dementia', because this is the term most commonly used and referred to within these wards. However, this is an umbrella term for a large number of different diseases that can cause or contribute to its onset. The most commonly recognised is Alzheimer's disease; however, there are many more (vascular dementia, Lewy Body, Parkinson's disease, frontotemporal, and the rarer types of dementia such as Creutzfeldt-Jakob's disease and Huntington's disease). It is recognised in deficits in cognition (thinking, remembering, and reasoning) and when these deficits represent a decline in cognitive functioning. It is also recognised in associated behavioural features, characterised by deterioration or changes in emotional control and social behaviour. Importantly, it is not a normal feature of ageing, and these cognitive and behavioural features must represent a significant decline in an individual's previous level of functioning, and impact on social functioning and daily living. These features are progressive; with deterioration inevitable. There are several established international criteria for the diagnosis of dementia, including the Diagnostic and Statistical Manual (DSM) of Mental Disorders and the International Classification of Diseases (ICD), which corresponds to a textbook form of knowledge.

As Ludwik Fleck (1979) tells us, textbooks embody just one version of scientific or medical knowledge. They provide a static picture of a condition, with little to indicate that these descriptions, and even their core, defining features, may be subject to debate or change over time. They typically omit features that are contested and shore up the often-indistinct and unclear borders of classifications, removing the uncertainties of scientific evidence. These textbook definitions can conceal and obscure the many different features associated with the large number of types and subtypes, and the diverse range of symptoms and features that can present in the individual. In dementia, these can include a diverse range of features, for example, visuo-perceptual symptoms (hallucinations), visual agnosias (difficulties with recognising faces or objects), apraxias (motor planning difficulties), Parkinsonism (tremor, slowed movements, changes in gait), to name but a few.

We can also view ongoing classificatory developments, such as the emergence of a range of prodromal categories, as attempts within the field to shore up these classificatory challenges. A key and recent shift in this classificatory framework for dementia has taken place in the publication of the fifth edition of the DSM diagnostic textbook, DSM-5 (American Psychological Association (APA) 2013), which produces the standard classifications of mental disorders used by mental health professionals (predominantly in the USA, but with a far wider influence). The goal of this diagnostic tool is to reflect current diagnostic 'consensus' within and across the clinical and research communities in the field of mental health. Within the most recent edition, the category 'Delirium, Dementia, Amnestic, and Other Geriatric Cognitive Disorders' (APA 2013) has transformed into the new category 'major neurocognitive disorder'. This category has also expanded to include earlier stages of cognitive impairment and decline, with mild cognitive impairment (MCI) recognised through the introduction of 'mild neurocognitive disorder' (APA 2013). These prodromal, preclinical, or 'predementia' categories describe and classify the point after normal aging and prior to the development of a major neurocognitive disorder, in which memory loss is present, but not at a level to meet the clinical criteria for the disorder (Petersen et al. 2001). However, these ongoing developments, in turn, lead to further fragmentation, variations and uncertainty in these diagnostic categories at clinical, scientific and regulatory levels (Moreira et al. 2009).

As we can see, within the nosographic category of dementia the ongoing clinical and biomedical explorations continue to reveal it to be more complex, less stable, and less firmly bounded entities than the original classifications implied. As Bowker and Star make clear in their examination of tuberculosis, 'The classification of the disease … does not stand alone; it is inserted into a shifting terrain of possible classification systems and cultural symbols' (2000: 173). As they suggest, these categories and classifications are highly variable and can be subject to considerable change and transformation over time.

The place of clinical entities within wider systems of knowledge (for example, dementia as a neurodegenerative disease, a mental health condition, or as a disability) and the ways in which these different systems are recognised and understood by different specialists, both locally (for example, within clinical gerontology, by neuroscience, or by community care practitioners) and globally (there will be variations in the local practices of recognition, for example, between UK memory clinics and neurologists in the USA), reflect their specific scientific and clinical specialisms and allegiances, which are all subject to change and transformation. Adjudicating and establishing the appropriate diagnosis, and its recognition and attribution to individuals, does not automatically entail a straightforward application of a predefined set of clinical criteria and parameters.

Importantly, 'dementia is a syndrome (a collection of symptoms) not a disease; it cannot be diagnosed, only recognised' (Manthorpe and Iliffe 2016: 5). As a syndrome (World Health Organisation (WHO) 1992), dementia is clinically recognised and assigned to an individual based on the observation and adjudication of a cluster of signs and symptoms. Specialist teams (gerontology, neurology and psychiatry) and clinics (memory clinics) typically employ a range of cognitive tests (across a range of domains), history taking (with patient and family), including history of function or deterioration, with a focus on the interaction between psychological tests and clinical judgement key features in the assembly and adjudication of dementia. Dementia is also a 'wastebasket' condition (Lock 2013), where diagnosis is by exclusion and involves a range of clinical tests to rule out other underlying clinical causes but also one that can 'be applied when nothing else fits' (Rosenhan 1975: 467). For individuals, the process of assessment and diagnosis within specialist clinics is typically lengthy and protracted, involving a large number of cognitive tests that can be distressing for patients, and is characterised by uncertainty (Manthorpe et al. 2013). The 'gold standard' diagnostic criteria is neuropathology; however, whether a diagnosis is achieved within the specialist clinic, the laboratory, or post-mortem at autopsy, standardisation remains elusive (Scheltens and Rockwood 2011). As Lock reminds us in her detailed exploration of the phenomenon of Alzheimer's disease, 'in short, it is a stubborn conundrum' (2016: 11).

A key response to this complexity and variation has been the 'repeated efforts over the years to refine the standardisation of the diagnosis both for use in the clinic and for epidemiological purposes' (Lock 2013: 54) through the use of biomarkers (neuroimaging (MRI, CT), cerebrospinal fluid (CSF), and genetic testing etc. Although these potential and emergent diagnostic technologies are typically currently limited to the domains of research, they have the potential to enter clinical services and may lead to further transformations in the diagnostic criteria and the clinical processes of assessment (Boenink 2016), reflecting more broadly long-standing expectations that technological and medical representation of underlying pathologies will replace clinical judgement (Featherstone et al. 2005).

Thus, 'dementia' exists in multiple versions, is produced and reproduced in multiple sites, and through multiple specialist and non-specialist, clinical, and biomedical frames, which are, in turn, further shaped by public policies and everyday cultural understandings. The recognition of these classificatory challenges and associated ongoing debates have taken place predominantly within the scientific and clinical fields, focussed on stabilising the condition for large-scale biomedical research and in understanding the underlying biomedical pathways. However, the impacts of the renewed interest within the wider public and policy spheres can be seen in the increasing focus placed on improving diagnosis rates, and this has manifested in the prioritisation of earlier diagnosis, the setting of diagnostic targets, and the establishment of specialist diagnostic clinics and memory assessment services, so called out-patient 'memory clinics' (in the UK) within the community. In parallel, there has been increasing debate about the efficacy of promoting clinical assessment and widespread screening for dementia and mild cognitive impairment and the impacts on individuals, families, and community services (LeCouteur et al. 2013). However, one key site where dementia as a clinical entity is assembled, adjudicated, recognised, and applied and where its consequences have been less recognised and understood is the acute hospital.

The significance of the acute setting for the recognition and attribution of dementia

The significance of the acute setting for these everyday processes of recognition and attribution of dementia and for the classification of older people cannot be understated. A significant number of people living with dementia have their first assessment when they are admitted to hospital with an acute condition (Holmes 1999). Following a hip fracture, of those living with dementia (40%), over a quarter (27%) received their diagnosis during their hospital admission (Holmes 1999). It is at once a site where it is increasingly recognised that a large number of people living with dementia will be located, but also a site (as we have explored in the previous chapter) where there is both invisibility and variable recognition. The acute ward is a site where there are complex interactions between dementia, the impacts of the acute admitting condition, and the ward setting itself, creating a site with potential for high levels of both under- and over-diagnosis.

Within the acute setting, although prevalence rates will differ by hospital and be dependent on their specific population, dementia is predominantly seen as an under-diagnosed condition due to a combination of underreporting and late diagnosis (National Audit Office 2007). Estimates suggest that in the UK, approximately 50% of those affected have not received a formal diagnosis in their medical records (Sampson et al. 2009, Goldberg et al. 2012, Russ et al. 2012). There are a range of potential reasons for this potential under-diagnosis (Koch and Iliffe 2010) or delayed diagnosis (Albert et al. 2011) of dementia, with much of this believed to be due to clinical teams not having the appropriate expertise (Koch and Iliffe 2010). This may be associated with barriers to diagnosis within primary care, such as issues of stigma and disclosure and uncertainty amongst clinicians about making this diagnosis (Koch and Iliffe 2010).

However, there are also likely to be many older people within the acute setting who may appear to ward staff to have dementia, but whose apparent cognitive decline may be associated with their hospital admission. There is a wide spectrum of other potential underlying causes of cognitive decline within the acute setting. There are high rates of delirium or sub-syndromal delirium within this acute population. With one screening study of a large cohort of older patients following an unplanned admission within an acute hospital setting (MAU) not only found a high prevalence of delirium (15.5%), but importantly identified high rates of undiagnosed (72%) delirium amongst this population (Collins et al., 2010). There are also high levels of co-morbid mental health (Goldberg et al. 2012) and alcohol-related brain damage (Gupta and Warner 2008) within this population.

Recognition and attribution of dementia within these wards

As discussed, we refer to '*dementia*', because this is the term that overwhelmingly reflects the everyday usage and recognition within these wards, with the major subtypes having very limited recognition. Within these wards, staff would typically talk of 'dementia', but would also (but less frequently) refer to

'Alzheimer's' which reflects wider public understandings (Hillman and Latimer 2017), while only occasionally referring to rarer subtypes. Local practices and understandings of a condition can have significant consequences, not only for individual patients, but also for shaping the practical recognition of the condition itself, and here we explore the ways in which these local processes have important consequences for older patients and for the work of these wards.

'Memory checks' at the bedside

The assessment of older patients where a diagnosis of dementia was suspected (or expected) occurred frequently within these wards. Although staff could make referrals to specialist medical and nursing teams, including gerontology, neurology and psychiatry (with dementia as a condition typically the domain of old age psychiatry in these hospitals), within these wards, requests to these specialities typically only occurred for cases that were viewed as particularly unusual or complex. As part of the admission process and the ongoing reviews and everyday assessments (both formal and informal) during bedside care of people living with dementia and older patients within these wards, staff typically focussed on assessing cognitive function, often with (as we have described earlier) an implicit expectation of identifying cognitive loss in older patients. The Mini-Mental State Examination (MMSE) referred to by staff as the 'mini-mental' is a well-recognised test designed to evaluate an older person's orientation, attention, memory, and language use across the domains of clinical and biomedical research, and the most visible and established diagnostic tool within these hospitals.

Over the course of our observations, although the 'mini-mental' was talked about and referred to, we did not see staff applying the standard MMSE test in practice. It was rare for any of the actual questions contained within the 'mini-mental' to form part of these assessments. Although this tool is described as a quick test to administer (taking ten minutes), this is considered a long time within these wards, and staff (across all specialisms and roles) typically relied on the use of single questions (sometimes variants of MMSE questions) at the bedside during what was often referred to by ward staff as a 'memory check' focussing on assessing orientation and memory during their often brief history taking at the bedside. During these 'checks', staff focussed on assessing cognitive features associated with the condition, primarily on memory loss in the abstract. Within these wards, cognition was always understood linguistically, and all assessments of the person focused on judgements of their interaction with staff and the ability to answer questions promptly and express themselves (for example by demonstrating reason or orientation) verbally.

We found that across these sites, these assessments were typically limited to a single, or a short series, of questions, from a limited repertoire heard again and again on these wards. These questions were delivered without thought for the specific context or the individual they were addressing, often appeared (to us and to the older person they were directed to) an unsuitable, incongruous and sometimes bizarre form of interrogation. This commonly included staff asking a patient confined within a bay or room without windows or a clock to state the time of day; asking a patient where they were (when they had just been woken up or recently been moved and had not been told of their location); or requirements that patients recall general knowledge, for example, historical dates (almost always related to significant dates in the world wars), name prominent political figures ('Who is the Prime Minister?') or state the age of members of the British Royal Family ('How old is the Queen?'). These questions rarely included any cultural considerations, any consideration that the person may simply not know the answer to the question, or consider that the question may bring back distressing experiences from their past.

> The medical team are with the man in bed 1. He does not have a diagnosis of dementia. They ask him about his cognitive state, asking him if he 'feels delirious?'. (I think it must be odd to be self-aware of this?) 'Are you hallucinating?' (Again, would self-awareness be possible?) and tell him that they are going to send him for 'a brain scan'. 'We are going to find out what's happening in your head to get you back on your feet.' After a few minutes, the patient tells the doctor that he trusts her. She tells him they need to do a memory test, and that this will involve ten questions. The questions include asking him what the time is. The doctor points out he is a couple of hours out. The patient responds that he has no way of knowing on the ward as there are no windows or clocks. She then asks him questions about the start of World War II.
>
> At the other side of the bay the Older Persons Specialist Nurse is doing a similar test with the patient in bed 9, whom she has just woken up to complete the test. As with the other memory test going on in this bay, this patient is fine until questioned about the time, which confuses him as he has no frame of reference. As he lies propped up by pillows on the bed, this nurse is leaning over the sidebar as she does the test, she has her face very close to his. she moves on to questions about the dates of World War II and the age of the Queen again. The nurse is talking in a clear loud voice, made doubly necessary as a neighbouring patient has begun to shave with a loud electric razor. At the end of the test she apologises for asking so many questions so soon after he had woken up, and reminds him that the doctor will be coming to see him soon. The facial expressions of this patient suggest he is slightly embarrassed and has found some of the questions challenging.
>
> (Site C day 2)

These approaches to assessments were routinely observed and although the questions about the world wars and the Queen are not part of the MMSE, they were consistently used by staff across these wards to assess capacity and categorise the patient. They reflected the cultures of recognition within these wards and the pervasive constructions of the generic 'elderly person' who is expected to have some cognitive loss. Regardless of actual age or background, all older patients were viewed by ward staff as having been born *c.*1920, closely followed the life of the Queen and the royal family, and would be happy to discuss what had happened to them and their families during violent global conflict. These stereotypes were consistent across staff specialisms and clinical teams, with these narrow constructions of the older person further informing the interpretation of the results of this assessment (or, more commonly, their response to one question), where a failure to respond as required, directed staff and signposted a potential diagnosis of dementia. Importantly, these approaches failed to consider or acknowledge the immediate and potentially temporary impacts of the person's acute admitting condition, often a traumatic event, on cognition and orientation.

Informal recognition of bays and cohorts of patients

We found that the attribution of who did and did not have dementia within these wards was typically made quickly by staff surveying their bays and at the bedside. Key factors in its attribution included judgements of their physical appearance (older patients) and behaviour (resistance to timetabled care, and behaviour viewed as disruptive, inappropriate, or transgressive) in response to the delivery of bedside care. These assessments were passed on and discussed with other team members during the everyday work of these wards and would be translated and recorded within the bedside records and team handover notes. These recording practices included 'd', 'D', 'dem', 'dementia?', 'query dementia' or '?dementia', diagnostic labels within these wards, even as a query, that once attached to an older person may not be questioned and could quickly assumed to be established.

We identified processes of contagion and spread in the recognition and application of this category. The established routine care practices believed to be appropriate for one group – people living with dementia – could quickly become attached to a wider group of older people within these wards. This could be exacerbated by common practices of zoning or 'corralling' patients who share specific attributes placed together within wards and bays. As we have already discussed, assigning beds by dependency (Roth and Eddy 1967) or to 'age grade' patients (Zerubavel 1979) within wards is a long-standing organisational practice and a persistent feature of ward cultures. Often this resulted in older people living with and without dementia cohorted side by side within bays and units. This could inform staff understandings of the population within specific bays and the wider ward during that shift and for individual patients throughout their admission. It was common for different staff within and entering a ward to have different views of an older patient's diagnosis, which could inform their placement within the ward, and their care. The example below comes from speaking to a range of staff working within a single bay over the course of an hour. The older patients within one large nine-bed bay were initially classified by ward staff as predominantly living with dementia; however, the Older Person's Nurse was not sure who had a diagnosis of dementia within the bay and the dementia care worker refuted this classification locating the patients with dementia in a different room within the unit:

> The Ward Sisters guide me to a closed-off bay of nine beds, all occupied by male patients. They tell me this is where the most patients with dementia have been admitted that morning (which is consistent with discussion in the unit's handover meeting that morning), and where I am best to make observations [...] I speak to the specialist Older Person's Nurse. She is only assigned to

> certain patients based on their age, admission and diagnosis and does not have access to the notes of patients to whom she is not assigned. None of the patients she is assigned to today has a formal diagnosis of dementia; she says this is unusual. Her tone of voice when discussing diagnosed dementia implies there may be more undiagnosed cases. I speak to one of the dementia care workers as she passes the bay and she confirms that that there are no diagnosed dementia patients on the bay, and only five on the whole of the unit today, and all are on the ladies' bays. She says that it can all change very quickly. She tells me the volume is always random, you cannot predict it and it can change very quickly. We discuss that there seem to be a small number of patients with a dementia diagnosis with the Nurse in Charge. Point out that in the handover meeting at the start of the shift it was acknowledged by the Matron that there were lots of patients with dementia who refuse care on this bay, and that she seemed to believe that people living with dementia were everywhere today.
>
> (Site C day 1)

Thus, the routine interactional practices and bedside care believed to be appropriate for people living with dementia could quickly become recognised and applied as standard care for a large and heterogeneous group of patients aged 65 years and over, but who were understood to be a homogeneous population with similar care needs within these bays and wards.

Categories and naming in the recognition of 'dementia'

Reductive understandings and recognition of categories of patients were visible in the everyday cultures of naming and labelling practices that pervaded everyday talk within these wards. Informal categories including 'feeders' and 'wanderers' were coupled with the designation of types of patients through categories of behaviour as 'climbers', and 'shouters', and broad descriptions of an individual's mental acuity as being 'confused', 'pleasantly confused', and the 'muddled'. Describing an older person as having 'confusion' was commonplace and widely used, an attribution that at once could be (and often was) viewed as unproblematic and requiring no further clinical investigations, but which could trigger an assessment for dementia.

The recognition and assessment of types of 'behaviour' dominated recognition of dementia in the person. For people living with dementia and older people within these wards, symptoms that could be associated with their admitting condition (for example, older people admitted with an infection or delirium can present with confusion, disorientation, agitation) or the impact of the ward environment itself and the restrictions placed upon the person during their admission, could potentially become recognised and interpreted as behavioural features of dementia and this categorisation could quickly become applied informally by ward staff to the person. These classes of patient were informed by the recognition of behaviour, typically described by staff as '*disruptive*', and viewed was inappropriate or transgressive of the rules of the ward in some way. Such behaviour became something understood by staff as a highly visible and dominant feature of a dementia diagnosis. However, being viewed as '*disruptive*' could quickly become an individual's principal identity within the context of these ward, with their dementia, or the assembled features recognised as dementia, overshadowing the person and their needs. Longer-term, chronic 'disruptive behaviour' could become a key feature overshadowing the person.

It was common for people who were calling out for attention, or visibly distressed within these wards to be disregarded (for example, as we have seen with Amanda in Chapter 2 and Sophie in Chapter 3). In some cases, this recognition could take the form of affection from staff, '*She's alright, she just likes a bit of a strop*' (site B day 15) and '*She does make me laugh though*' (site D day 8). However, when people were so distressed that this had negative impacts on other patients, interrupted the timetabled work of these wards, or when they were able to leave the bedside and viewed as having the potential to 'wander' or 'abscond', they were likely to receive the most attention from staff. These new identities were viewed negatively and circulated the ward: '*he is a puncher*' (site C day 2), '*she is a hitter*' (site E day 5). Such classes of people were typically approached at the bedside with caution; for staff, however, there was always an underlying fear and expectation (often with good reason) that a patient could respond physically. Some, usually male (although not always), patients living with dementia would be approached by staff in pairs, or a male member of staff would be asked to approach them, regardless of the person's present mood or behaviour.

This category of patient was also likely to be confined to their bed or bedside, or moved to side rooms, where the additional isolation could increase their distress, boredom, loneliness, and dependency. This could lead to the person being supervised more closely, which could, in turn, cause further distress, anxiety, and prompt these wards to initiate organisational disciplinary processes. These processes, known as 'enhanced care', but typically referred to within these wards as 'specialing', where a patient is 'specialed', takes the form of closer supervision and restriction of the person. The most common and visible sign of this category of patient is the presence of one-to-one care, an agency carer or student nurse tasked with sitting at the 'specialed' persons bedside. There are also less visible, but equally powerful bureaucratic means of recognising this category of patient within these wards, most notably the Deprivation of Liberty Safeguarding order, leading to their recognition as the 'DoLS patient'. We will discuss these strategies and their impacts in more detail within Chapters 6 and 7.

These understandings of dementia as a category led to the 'dementia patient' being recognised in ways that emphasised them as deviant and disruptive within the ward. Once a patient was recognised in this way, their attempts to assert autonomy and decision-making were typically interpreted by staff within these wards as a further expression of their dementia diagnosis, attributed to 'confusion', cognitive loss and loss of the person. Non-verbal, or embodied, communication was not recognised as such, but typically understood and viewed by staff as resistive, disruptive, inappropriate, or transgressive behaviour to be managed and limited within these wards. Such approaches effaced the complexity of the range of symptoms associated with the condition, and the wide array of potential impacts of the ward on the person.

Stickiness of the label and recognition of dementia

Dementia appeared to overshadow as a default diagnosis for many older people (both formally and informally applied) within these wards, particularly if their admitting condition reduced their current capacity or mobility. This had the potential to reduce opportunities for the recognition of competing classifications at the boundaries of these disease entities such as other mental health conditions and delirium, or key features of the admitting condition such as pain or other acute conditions (as we will see with Rebecca shortly). We found that it also overshadowed patients' attempts to communicate other immediate care needs such as hunger, thirst or continence (as we have described in Chapter 3, with Sophie). The 'stickiness' (Rosenhan 1979) of this label, and the ways in which these behavioural features or embodied forms of communication visible at the bedside, could inform perceptions of the older person, with the potential to shape understandings and responses to them throughout their admission.

As we have discussed, a person's diagnosis of dementia was rarely the reason for their admission to these wards. The primary cause of an admission was likely to be an infection, most frequently of the urinary tract, or a fracture following a 'fall'. We observed that within these wards, potentially significant (and well-recognised) symptoms and risk factors associated with these admitting conditions could quickly be overshadowed, and instead become recognised as features of their dementia diagnosis or signs of undiagnosed dementia. The recognition of what ward staff would typically label as 'confusion', 'refusal', or 'aggression' would frequently be interpreted by ward teams as key features of dementia. This often meant that staff did not explore other potential causes associated with their admitting condition.

Rebecca was admitted following a seizure and was initially assessed by the team as 'resisting care' and having 'undiagnosed dementia'. During this time, her behaviour and responses to her admission fluctuated dramatically; at times, she angrily refused meals or argued with other patients, while at other times she would happily make jokes and laugh with staff. However, this developed into hallucinations and she had regular hallucinatory conversations at the bedside. During the taking of the patient's history by a junior member of the medical team, her hallucinations were apparent. However, in response, he focussed on talking to her in an increasingly loud voice and slowly enunciating his words, emphasising his recognition and assessment that her behaviour was related to dementia and cognitive impairment. It was only many days later that this behaviour, or 'symptoms', became recognised as a feature of her acute admitting condition and she was diagnosed with an infection and delirium (hyperactive delirium, which is defined by agitation, restlessness, and hallucinations, in comparison to hypoactive delirium, which is characterised by drowsiness and withdrawal).

> Rebecca has returned to her hallucinatory conversation, turned to the left and speaking in an engaged tone of voice, changing pitch as if having a really gossipy conversation with a close friend. Her tray table has been cleared, and she now has only bananas left upon it, in front of her and easily within reach. A junior member of the medical arrives at her bedside, asking her how she is.

> Rebecca, now talking in a very high and loud voice, tells the doctor she is fine. The junior doctor attempts to take Rebecca's medical history but does not get far as her answers are unrelated or incoherent. He then asks Rebecca if she can remember why she came to the hospital and she answers excitably but about something unrelated. He explains to her that she 'had a fit', and tries to establish if she has had any history of this previously. He is doing the 'Englishman abroad' trick of repeating the same question, but in an increasingly slow and loud tone of voice. Rebecca continues to answer in full sentences, but all unrelated to the questions. He establishes that she does not seem aware of what day it is, where she is, nor that she is in a hospital. He explains that she is going to have to stay in the ward for a little bit longer. She was originally set to be discharged yesterday, when she was more alert and coherent and seems to be deteriorating in both function and cognition over this admission.
>
> (Site D day 4)

This was a common feature of our observations within these wards, where screening for dementia (this was carried out by a wide range of individuals, teams and specialisms) was part of history-taking on admission. This was a setting where older people could be quickly assigned an informal diagnosis of dementia, rather than other forms of temporary impairment (behavioural or cognitive) symptomatic of treatable acute medical conditions. These processes of assessment and recognition of dementia could overshadow the potential for other underlying causes. In the case of Rebecca, such assumptions could be (and were) cleared up quite simply, by the team speaking to family members later that same morning:

> Rebecca has gone quiet and subdued at this point, she is no long shouting. Her family have called to let the team know they are on their way and while on the phone they confirm that Rebecca is not deaf, as had been suspected and recorded in her notes, and that her behaviour is common for her when she has had infections in the past. They tell the team Rebecca will 'typically snap out of it' and have full cognitive capacity again once the infection has been treated, with no lasting impairment. A pair of foundation year doctors in the corridor are discussing how surprised they are at the vividness of her hallucinations and confusion, they did not know people could hold full hallucinatory conversations with multiple people.
>
> (Site D day 4)

However, not all patients have family available to advocate for them as a person (and families were not always consulted) nor to challenge the classifications of the ward. For many, the assumed diagnosis of dementia would inform their subsequent care.

Recognition of the impacts of the ward environment

Observing these wards for long periods during and across shifts, over many weeks, in many ways gives the researcher a position of privilege that ward staff could not share. The assignment of ward staff to different bays from one shift to another was usual practice and this meant that staff typically were not able to follow the experiences of an individual patient over time and across their admission. They only typically experienced episodic and short interactions at the patient's bedside during task-based timetabled care at specific points within a shift. This meant they were not able to witness the impacts of the admission, or indeed the often-powerful impacts of the organisation of the work of the ward and the delivery of bedside care on older people and people living with dementia over time.

We found that just by passing a patient's bed, the doorway of the bay they were admitted to or the entrance of a single occupancy room, the ward team could generate powerful feelings of isolation, distress, and fear in older patients. This was the point when patients often called out and asked for support and for help, with what was often a pressing and urgent need. However, in the context of these ward cultures, the expected pace of work and focus on individual staff caseloads and timetables, passing staff typically did not respond to people's cries for help, nor respond even when the person was clearly expressing a pressing need, for example, for personal care, continence care, pain, or reassurance. The organisational mandates of these wards emphasised the prioritisation of individual caseloads and the completion of the timetables, which were powerfully felt by staff.

However, the majority of ward staff did not see or recognise that by not responding, but instead walking by, this often increased the levels of distress felt by the person in question. This often culminated in them attempting to leave (to 'wander' or 'abscond') the bedside or the ward. Staff typically did not see or recognise these impacts, because they had already moved on, leaving it to other members of staff (it was often not clear, particularly within some of these wards, who this would be) to respond. Within one ward (site D), we discussed this with members of the therapy team, who paused and spent a few minutes observing the many beds arranged to face inwards towards the typically busy nursing station at the centre of the bay. The members of the therapy team were shocked when they observed that simply by repeatedly passing a patient's bedside, and not responding and ignoring a patient who called out or asked for assistance, they had been inadvertently causing high levels of distress, triggering sobbing, repeated calls for help, and attempts to leave the bedside for that person throughout their admission. In the example below, a patient described by staff as being 'easily agitated' is placed in a bed facing a busy corridor with lots of staff constantly passing by, and she becomes increasingly distressed as the day progressed.

> At the start of the day's observation a member of the dementia specialist team sees me in the corridor and recommends I observe a particular bay, where one patient has been quite agitated all morning. Mary is 90 years old, and has been admitted from a care home. She is in the care home temporarily while her husband recovers in hospital from a stroke. The home has admitted her to the medical assessment unit because of her behaviour. She has no medical condition. However, initial attempts to discharge Mary have been cancelled as the care home will not accept her back. Her 'agitation' has escalated throughout her admission. Staff are angry with the home, as it is more

appropriate for her, better resourced and they need the bed for other patients with medical issues. The bay Mary is on is an overflow bay only used when the unit is over-capacity. The other patients on the bay include a patient going through alcohol withdrawal and a young woman on suicide watch. Mary is the only patient with dementia. She is in bed and is shouting in a very high-pitched voice that is difficult to understand. Initially, the entrance to the bay is locked due to the other patients attempting to leave, and staff have to knock to enter. Mary shouts whenever anybody comes through the door.

Staff do not immediately respond when Mary shouts. When two nurses go to her bedside to look at equipment at her bedside they do not speak to her. It is only when Mary speaks to them, pointing her finger at them that they acknowledge and respond, 'Hello young lady! What's the matter?' Mary settles when they have spoken to her.

Just after 15:00 the healthcare assistant comes back on the bay. She has been escorting another patient for a cigarette. Mary shouts 'EXCUSE ME' at the nurse in charge. She responds, 'Two minutes sweetie' as she leaves the bay. Mary begins to shout 'HELLO!' whenever anybody passes her bed, which is located right next to the now open ward door, which faces a busy corridor. It is not possible to pass the door or enter or exit the ward without passing Mary. She is in full view of the corridor and calls out whenever anybody passes by. When staff respond to her she smiles a full beaming smile that the nurse mentioned to me earlier, but when they ignore her she gets upset, causing the lady in the neighbouring bed to attempt to reassure and calm her. It sounds as if Mary is crying, but this may just be her high-pitched intonation. The lady in the next bed keeps telling Mary to try and keep calm, reminds her that her family are coming and not to get upset.

By now (it is 15:25) Mary asks every passing member of staff if she can go home, it sounds as if she is pleading, it is upsetting to hear. In the corridor the senior nurses are discussing the need to free up beds. I hear the nurse in charge of Mary's bay question why Mary has been left there. At 15.30 Mary begins to call out for somebody to come and see her. The nurse tells her she needs to do some jobs then will come and talk to her, leaving the lady in the next bed to speak to her. Mary kicks off her bedsheet.

A social care worker comes on to the bay for another patient, but they are away from their bed. Mary shouts 'EXCUSE ME' to her. The social worker, who is dressed like she works at the hospital, responds 'Sorry I'm not staff, I don't work here' and leaves the bay. The nurse in charge walks back on to the bay. As she passes Mary's bed she again shouts, asking if she can go home. This continues throughout the afternoon. Mary calls out every time anybody passes her bed, which is the only way to get on or off the bay. When ignored she kicks the sheets off her bed, and has begun to whimper whenever she is ignored. Only the lady in the neighbouring bed responds to this. It is extremely upsetting to hear Mary whimpering in her bed and I speak to the nurse and she acknowledges to me that this is not the right place for Mary to be left. She is not happy about Mary being here, Mary is medically well and should not be stuck on an overflow assessment unit.

> At 15.45 a nurse and healthcare assistant pass Mary's bed. 'WON'T SOMEBODY HELP ME', she shouts. After she settles, the next few passes do not seem to bother her (at least not as overtly). Staff at the station do not seem to bother her, only people passing her bed. The staff at the station have begun to acknowledge her, but only to the extent to offering sympathetic 'aws' and 'ahs' when Mary calls out.
>
> Except for a 10-minute period when one of the specialist dementia staff comes to talk to her, Mary continues to sporadically shout for help throughout the afternoon. At one point the Older Person's Specialist Nurse and a pharmacist talk about Mary while she calls out to them behind her. They can't get her regular medications, and at the same time are still waiting for social services to 'sort themselves out' and find somewhere that Mary can be discharged to.
>
> (Site C day 13)

The more these actions occurred over a shift or across a patient's admission, the more unremarkable the behaviour becomes as a feature of their dementia or who the person is, and, in turn, the less urgent the responses from staff become. For example, shouting becomes recognised by staff as a symptom of 'confusion' and 'dementia', rather than potentially a feature of the acute admitting condition or an underlying and potentially urgent care need. Rarely was the reason or intent of the patient's actions be investigated or discussed with the patient, beyond the 'aws' and 'ahs' above and rhetorical platitudes such as 'Where are you going?' and 'What's wrong, darling?'. The heterogeneous patient is instead overshadowed by deeply entrenched understandings of the recognition of dementia and the scrutiny of patients during the performance of bedside care.

These patterns were commonplace within these wards. When the impacts on patients of such common, everyday actions and interactions were hidden from staff by the organisation cultures and pace of the work of these wards, the impacts of the more complex and nuanced cascade of interactions and invisibilities on people living with dementia became obscured further still. It was as if the person living with dementia was viewed as an island, existing in isolation within these wards, unaffected by the social world in which they involuntarily find themselves. Rarely, if ever, was there any consideration that many of these responses could in fact be generated by the ward environment, a reaction to the organisation and delivery of routine bedside care, and care practices within these wards. The potential complex and powerful interactions between the hospital admission, the organisation and delivery of care, and the acute admitting condition and additional co-morbid conditions such as dementia, were rarely recognised or acknowledged within these wards.

Constructing dementia as high dependency

People living with dementia were often very capable of many forms of self-care during their admission, including eating meals, walking independently and going to and from the bathroom. This independence was typically not recognised, and often denied by the organisational cultures of these wards, which expected people living with dementia to need support at mealtimes, to be unable to walk independently, and to be considered to be high risk of further injuries (particularly of 'falls'), with often presumed incontinence. A patient who had been living independently at home becomes 'high dependency' or 'dependent' on admission, their actions then defined by organisational perceptions of risk rather than personal agency and ability.

Importantly, once a person was regarded within these wards as having increased dependency, it often became a self-fulfilling label. Older people and people living with dementia were typically less able to adapt or to make their needs known within this environment, Thus, people categorised as having dementia and thus high dependency were cared for at the bedside in ways that could result in them losing further skills and independence. A patient who 'wet themselves' in their bed as a result of being told repeatedly by staff to stay in bed could become quickly classified as 'incontinent'; or spilling food on themselves and their bed because ward staff insist that they eat a bowl of breakfast cereal or soup while lying in their bed (which is more difficult than staff seemed to assume) could become viewed a 'feeder'; a patient who stumbles at the bedside as a result of equipment placed around them becomes 'at risk of falls'. This labelling also led to greater scrutiny of the individual and the requirement by staff that they become aligned and adhere more closely to the routines of these wards, a tightening and contraction of their timetables of care, creating more opportunity for further resistance to care, which we will explore in more detail within the following chapters.

This had a further impact on shaping ward staff understandings of dementia and led to routine practices of care that limited opportunities for people living with dementia to rehabilitate and increase their independence. For ward staff, requiring help with eating meals and not being able to eat independently was viewed as a key feature of the condition. People were often identified by staff as 'feeders' (i.e. that they needed spoon feeding), even if they demonstrated during other shifts that they could eat independently or with minimal support. Ward staff across sites approached people at the bedside with the instruction '*We are going to feed you*' (site B day 4) and discussed individual patients with other ward staff '*I am going to feed x*' (site D day 11), '*Can he feed himself?*' (site B day 12) and '*We are feeding him first?*' (site A day 15). While this could arguably be viewed as a small linguistic tic, 'feeding' emphasises the lack of agency in the individual. People living with dementia, as in the case of Peter below, were often very capable of eating a meal without support. These assumptions about dependency could often be relatively good-natured, as in the example below; however, it does limit the agency of an otherwise capable patient:

> The nurse tells Peter to 'Stay where you are … you will miss it [lunch]'. Peter asks for a paper. The nurse responds, telling Peter 'If I can I can go down and get you one … it will get you through the afternoon', 'Yes it gets a bit boring', says Peter. The nurse turns to another and announces, 'He's hungry!', 'We are going to feed you', the other responds.
>
> (Site B day 4)

Peter, on other occasions during his admission, ate his meals independently. He wanted to read the newspaper and was able to provide droll quips to the ward team when in conversation with them, drawing laughs and displaying an acute awareness of his surroundings. However, within the ward his diagnosis of dementia overrode this. This classification meant he was recognised as a person who required 'feeding', rather than a patient who could be left to eat their meal. He was at once a person within the organisation of the ward, independent during informal interactions, but not within the formal bedside routines of the institution.

These assumptions about a patient's dependence in the context of accomplishing everyday tasks had a wider impact on how individuals with dementia were viewed and classified by staff. It influenced their wider understandings of the capacity, autonomy, independence, and the ability of people living with dementia to make decisions, and, in turn, impacting on all aspects of their care and potential for recovery. Here Deborah talks about her frustration at the way the ward underestimated her mother's independence, in terms of both her ability to make choices and also in the reduction of her mobility. She believed that such assumptions of high dependency as being an inevitability in people living with dementia were a deeply embedded feature of the culture on these wards:

DEBORAH: 'My mum after that length of time, being in that ward, I have to say was fed up, frustrated, and couldn't wait to go home, to be listening to her own music, be surrounded by people that she wanted to be around with, mainly me, doing her personal care and stuff and also most importantly she just wanted her independence back, her mobility. Yes she had to use machinery but she wanted to be, if she wanted to sleep she could sleep, if she wanted to listen to music she could listen, she could look out at her garden and yes you know have to adhere for risks and everything but she was so much better going home. That length of time in there, her muscle tone, if she hadn't been there her mobility might not have gone down so quickly, she might have had a little bit more time to use the equipment but we did have an amazing day where the occupational therapist and the physios came and everyone came and they said she can't walk and she proved that she could walk across the room and it was, sorry. [becomes very emotional and tearful] It was amazing. Sorry. I just need a minute that's all'.

(February 2019)

One of the key expectations informing understandings of dementia within these wards was that the person's life following discharge from the hospital would be limited. This was reflected in staff discussions on the condition. When talking to ward staff on breaks they would be sympathetic to and have empathy for their patients, but in black humour expressed their powerlessness, that they felt they could not do much to help them. Many expressed that they would not like to grow 'that old' themselves, or that if they had a diagnosis of dementia to 'take me outside and shoot me', or similar sentiments (as we have seen earlier in this chapter).

Ward expectations and the dismissal of a formal diagnosis

For some patients, their formal diagnosis of dementia could quickly be dismissed by ward staff, particularly if they did not conform to their expectations of who was a 'dementia patient'. By not meeting the archetype of the older 'dementia' patient routinely recognised within these wards, these people could find their diagnosed dementia denied, which impacted on the care provided to them.

During our series of consultations with people living with dementia to discuss our emerging analysis, many people in their 50s and early 60s who were living with dementia (Young Onset Dementia) described that their hospital admissions was where their diagnosis was questioned or denied by hospital staff. For example, Paul (pseudonym), who received a diagnosis of dementia (mixed Alzheimer's and Vascular Dementia) when he was 50 years old (Young Onset Dementia), described his recent hospital admission. He recalls being continually told by the ward staff caring for him that 'You don't look like you've got dementia' and 'You can't have Alzheimer's!'

PAUL: 'Well I was actually told a few times, well I still get told, how well I look, yes you can remember so you can't have Alzheimer's, and various things like that but a lot of the problem is public in general and staff in hospitals who should know better is that it's not just about memory, it's a lot of other things get affected as well so you can't judge someone's dementia progression on their memory.'

(February 2019)

He found that this powerfully influenced his care. Staff, who he expected 'should know better', judged that he had better cognitive abilities and capabilities, and presumed that he did not need support, for example with choosing meals from the menu, or need help finding the bathroom. He felt 'There's a lot of things that they don't take into account and there's a lot of things that they make misconceptions about as well'.

PAUL: 'The last time I was in hospital, I think it was after a stroke I had and people were more interested, the staff were more interested or seemed to be more interested in my dementia diagnosis rather than what I'd come in for and they were saying things like you don't look like you've got dementia? Well what does dementia look like? I probably also didn't look like I'd had a stroke, what does a person look like when they've had a stroke? So that seemed to matter much more than the actual treatment which was a bit worrying but then they'd also make assumptions that I couldn't hear, because I had dementia, and they'd speak louder to me, they'd also give me too many choices so then my stock answer then is no, so I was refusing meals then because and they were just okay, you're not hungry and take it away and nothing else and if I walked into the bathroom and walked out again then they took it that I'd looked after myself, cleaning wise and I hadn't. I walked in and didn't know what to do so walked out again. So there's a lot of things that they don't take into account and there's a lot of things that they make misconceptions about as well and they just see the dementia and not the person most of the time.'

(February 2019)

Discussion

Clinical conditions such as dementia are socially mediated. Diseases, conditions, and syndromes do not appear complete and fully realised in the body, or present themselves self-evidently to biomedical research, medical practitioners, or to clinical teams at the bedside. The work of diagnosis, of naming and claiming, requires the work of recognition, description, and interpretation of features in the body. Importantly, this is accomplished through socially organised work. The laboratory and the specialist clinic (such as the memory clinic) are important sites for knowledge production, where the collaborative work between experts, between and across disciplines, initiate, develop, and sustain understandings of disease categories and classes. In these wards, we observed the ways in which the very local sites (and the non-specialists within them) constitute a key location where the category dementia is produced and reproduced in the practical recognition during the delivery of routine bedside care.

There is nothing to suggest that the clinical category of dementia and the work that goes into classifying and treating them do not reflect actual biomedical disease in the body, the impacts of dementia on the person are well established; rather, within this chapter we wish to show the ways in which the category itself is subject to interpretation, in ways that can have powerful consequences for individuals. This ongoing work of recognition of the category 'dementia' is a fluid and ongoing social process, and within these wards it reflects a range of clinical and personal expertise, and understandings shaped within these ward cultures. Within these wards, dementia was a far more public, taken-for-granted classification applied to large numbers of older patients at the bedside. However, these classifications have consequences, and should be made with caution. A diagnosis of dementia represents 'a critical legitimation for institutionalisation' (Cohen 1998: 33) and thus has the potential to have significant implications for individuals which will inform their life chances and opportunities.

5 Tightening of the timetables and the organisation of bedside care

Introduction

Timetabled routines, and the 'task-list system' (Menzies Lyth 1959: 65) as a mode of coordinating the work of the hospital ward and the delivery of bedside care within them, has a long tradition (Stanton and Schwartz 1954, Caudill 1958, Coser 1962, Roth and Eddy 1967, Zerubavel 1979). Julius Roth, in an examination of the rehabilitation hospitals in the middle of the last century (1963), identified the competing timetables and their impacts. Patients were almost universally anxious to go home at the earliest opportunity, and viewed treatment almost more in terms of how it affected their pathway home, than in terms of clinical improvements. Conversely, Roth observed that staff within the institution had very different concerns, focussed on tasks and treatments and the pressures in establishing and maintaining the repeated procedures of the ward (1963: 22).

Importantly, we found that these organising principles and priorities seemed to have changed little from these earlier descriptions of ward life. Here we focus on the daily timetables of bedside work within these contemporary wards, governed by rigid, task-based timetables, that organised, shaped, and dominated the delivery of everyday care at the bedside (Featherstone et al. 2019). These organisational strategies demonstrate an institutional commitment to the systematic and standardised delivery and recording of care; however, they also powerfully shaped cultures within these wards through the production and reproduction of ward priorities, expectations of pace, mandated order of delivery, and informed what was considered valid work at the bedside. We found little to suggest their adaption to meet the needs of people living with dementia within them. Instead, these processes directed staff attention towards delivering a highly structured and restricted repertoire of recognised bedside care that reflected an archetypal and outmoded construct of the acute patient and their needs.

These organisational mandates shaped the work of these wards, increasing the visibility of some types of work as constituting essential care, which, in turn, diminished the visibility of (and potential for) other types of care, care needs, and patients. Importantly, we observed that these approaches appeared to exclude and devalue work that could not be easily quantified, measured, or recorded within the current systems, work that has been crudely described as 'compassionate' and 'person-centred' care. This highly skilled work requires learnt expertise, flexibility, responsiveness, and, often, a slow pace. This work is required to provide appropriate bedside care for vulnerable patients, but it cannot easily be quantified or mandated within rigid task-based structures. This is particularly observable for people living with dementia, who typically retain their own timetables and schedules and could not easily adapt to the highly structured care required by the organisational practices of these wards.

These routinised organisational practices produced fragmentation of care at the bedside, meaning ward staff delivered identical tasks (there was very little variation within and across sites) or 'rounds' of care, to many bedsides in a typically rigid order. This thus reduced opportunities for uninterrupted or significant time to be spent with individual patients, who, in turn, received their care from many different people arriving at the bedside to complete various 'tasks'. This approach to care increased the potential for detachment and reduced opportunities to see the person and their individual needs. We found that the more this bedside care work was distributed across a large number of small identical tasks and interactions to be completed and recorded, the more the accomplishment of the routine itself became the focus. We found that the patient, particularly people living with dementia, could become viewed as 'a potential source of disruption, added labour, and disturbance' (Roth and Eddy 1967: 49) in the drive to deliver the timetabled work within shifts. Within these wards, completing each aspect of the timetable, recording it, and moving on to the next patient in their bay, and then on to the next task, became the primary organisational concern. Thus, staff attention was driven by the desire to fulfil the inflexible and repetitive routines of these wards in order to meet the demands of the wider organisation.

This was reflected in the widespread underlying awareness of surveillance amongst staff that we observed, that falling behind was not to be tolerated and failing to meet the expectations of the timetable within a shift was not permissible and viewed as a significant personal shortcoming, visible to their team (and to the following team taking over the next shift) and the wider organisation. We too felt the constant 'tension, distress and anxiety' (Menzies Lyth 1959: 45) amongst ward staff, which was particularly intense during predictable points in the shift timetable (most notable during the second half of a day shift, but this could also be at points where external competing timetables, such as the external schedules of the medical team or auxiliary or catering teams, entered these wards), when it was usual for staff to feel additional pressure, that their timetable was slipping, or for the organisation of care to break down completely. The threat of the potential for 'falling behind' was routinely observable; patterns described by staff as 'coming in waves' (site B day 3), were well recognised and a regular topic of discussion in break rooms.

Importantly, these organisational mandates in themselves were, somewhat paradoxically, the main contributor to the breakdown of the timetables within these wards. These organisational pressures could lead to staff becoming increasingly focussed on delivering quantified tasks that must be recorded within bedside records. This reliance on routine unsurprisingly informed their replication of familiar interactions that could be (and were) delivered in the same way across the many bedsides with little adaption to the individual within it (we will explore this in more detail in the next chapter), typically triggered powerful somatic responses in people living with dementia (including resistance and refusal of care). As staff felt the timetable to be escaping them, these wards became increasingly pressurised, with the requests and needs of patients that fell outside any recognition of the organisational mandates of their 'appropriate tasks' (Roth and Eddy 1967: 40), became viewed as a patent's 'whims', which were increasingly inaccessible and invisible to them and were discouraged or ignored.

Restoring and repairing the timetables through increased pace, priorities, rigidity, and patterns of compulsive repetition at the bedside, was a key feature of the work on these wards during almost every shift. However, these approaches could rapidly generate patterns of contagion. The strategies of increased tightening of focus, rigidity of order, and repetition of aspects of the timetables, and an accelerated pace of bedside care, were all likely to generate significant stress and distress amongst everyone (both patients and staff) within these wards, which could spread across cohorts of patients and within teams, and transfer between patients and staff at the bedside. As the pace of work escalated, this could generate further activity and noise within these wards, which was associated with further distress (signalled by the sounds of buzzers triggered by bedside call buttons, machine alarms, and cries for support) across a wider group of patients and increasingly rigid and reactive cycles of care by staff as their timetables appeared to break down.

Once an individual or team felt that their timetables had broken down, care could quickly transition into approaches at the bedside that responded reactively, concentrating on highly visible care needs, and containing what they viewed as imminent patient risk. This could also lead to staff working at cross-purposes, team members repeating care at the same bedside, the increasing use of containment, restriction, and restraint (which we will explore in more detail later within Chapter 7) and for the care needs of silent and still patients to become invisible (as we have seen previously in Chapter 3). These habitual patterns within the life of these wards also powerfully shaped ward cultures, where praising the pace and volume of work, seeing the ward as like being in a 'war zone', could become markers of team identity and solidarity, but also demonstrated their significant distress to the wider institution.

Timetables and their impacts on people living with dementia

We have discussed (within the previous chapter) that observing these wards for long periods during and across shifts, over consecutive days and weeks, in many ways gave us a position of privilege that staff could not share. It was the usual practice for ward staff to be assigned to different bays and to have little continuity with their patients from one shift to another. This meant they were typically unable to follow the experiences of an individual patient over time nor across their admission. The structures of timetabled care also meant they were typically restricted to only experience short, high-volume, episodic, and repetitive task-based interactions at each patient's bedside, across each and every shift. Staff were rarely able to see the impacts of timetabled care on individual patients and people living with dementia over time.

It was common for a person living with dementia to have many underlying and often urgent physical needs (including personal care, continence care, thirst, hunger, and pain management) during their admission which were all recognised within the timetabled tasks of bedside care (although these needs could be problematic if requested outside of the designated points in the timetable). During our observations, it was apparent that they also experienced significant emotional distress (this included, for example, fear, loneliness, frustration, and despair). People living with dementia would frequently express fears about where they were, what was happening to them, and when their admission would end. A key (and understandable) anxiety was not knowing when they were going home, whether they would be able to leave and go home, and even if they still had a home. Other causes of anxiety, which were often invisible to staff but highly visible to us as observers, included not knowing where valuable personal items such as purses, handbag or wallets were, or fearing the loss (or presumed theft) of valuables such as jewellery or watches. People also became distressed at not wearing their own underwear, pyjamas, clothes, or slippers. In addition, a person's anxiety about where they were and what was happening to them, or what was happening to their home, family or pets could also quickly heighten and accelerate, if the unfamiliarity of their experiences increased in any way.

For many of the people we observed, these experiences and feelings were often difficult to communicate verbally, and instead became visible as a bodily manifestation (this can be seen in the example below, where Gareth's distress is embodied, sitting rigid in the chair, his arms tightly folded across his chest, hands clasped, wringing a tissue in his hand). We found that such signs of underlying anxiety were observable in every person living with dementia at some stage during their admission. Because we could both follow ward teams and patients over time, we were able to see that without early and prompt recognition and attention, these underlying care needs could quickly become more entrenched experiences of distress. However, these experiences could become recognised as a feature of their dementia (resistance to timetabled care, and behaviour viewed as disruptive, inappropriate, or transgressive in response to routine bedside care) and, as such, considered unremarkable within this setting.

Here the ward team deliver a large number of short task-based interactions, forming rounds of care to six men within a bay, but had few opportunities to spend uninterrupted or significant time with them. The organisational priorities of the timetabled order of the delivery of bedside care mean they are unable to recognise Gareth's underlying and increasingly urgent needs. This has consequences for both Gareth and the team that continue throughout this shift. Following the shift handover, the morning routines involved attending each bedside in succession (from bed 1 to bed 6) to provide personal care, a fresh change of clothes, stripping and changing all the beds, and helping these men to either sit up in bed or to sit in the bedside chair ready for breakfast. It was usual across these wards for the team to try to do this before the breakfast trolley arrived, bringing with it the competing timetable of the catering team. The bay team (a nurse and healthcare assistant) were attending a bedside together as a 'double' (two people were required to support the person) behind the curtain delivering personal care (washing, dressing and stripping and changing the bed) to a patient living with dementia who appeared to be minimally conscious (he was later identified as having a brain aneurysm following an accident at home). Gareth, who also has a diagnosis of dementia, is in the next bed and pulls at the curtain dividing them, telling the team 'I want to go home'. They admonish him for interrupting and return their focus on the immediate task behind the curtain. When this task is accomplished, they do not return to Gareth; instead they move on to the next task to meet the demands of the timetable.

> It is 7.45 a.m. and the bay team (healthcare assistant and nurse) stride to the bedside of the man in bed 5 and say to him 'Morning! … Just a little wash, my love.' The sheets are all rumpled and have ended at the bottom of the bed, he is lying in an odd position and doesn't move, his eyes are closed, and he seems to respond to them, although no words can be distinguished, this seems to be a general grumbling sound. They close the curtains around him and talk to him as they work. As they do this, Gareth, who is wearing hospital pyjamas and sitting in his chair at the neighbouring bedside, pulls back the curtains dividing them. The healthcare assistant pulls it back, but pokes her head out and explains to Gareth (in a slightly exasperated tone) that he needs to leave the curtain. He replies 'I want to go home'. She draws the curtains and they continue to talk to the man in bed 5 as they work on his body. 'It's just so we can get you all nice and fresh.' They are hidden behind the privacy curtain, but, in response, it sounds as though there is a scuffle and he is lashing out at them as they tell him firmly 'NO'.

With the team occupied, Gareth repeatedly attempted to get up from his chair, walk, and leave the bedside. However he becomes extremely frustrated because he has no strength and cannot stand for long. The team focus their attention on completing the immediate tasks at the other bedside, which seems to increase their anxiety and stress because this is not straightforward (there are sounds of a struggle behind the curtains). As they do this, they (and other ward staff passing in the corridor) repeatedly give Gareth clear instructions to sit down and remind him that he is in hospital:

> Gareth starts to get up from the bedside chair, pushing himself up into a standing position. He looks very determined and stands up by pushing down using the side arms on his chair and by resting his hands on his trolley, which is on wheels and looks very unstable. He looks very unsteady and his body is shaking from the effort, but has a very focussed and determined expression. The team are still behind the curtain and what sounds like a struggle: 'We are just putting your t shirt on … NO!' 'I know, we are just putting your t shirt on.' I check on Gareth. The nursing team have previously told him he is not able to walk, but he tells me that he wants his 'Zimmer', his walking frame, which is at the end of the bed and out of reach. At this point, the healthcare assistant comes out from behind the curtain with a large arm full of soiled

sheets and emphasises very firmly to him: 'You can't get up. You are not good on your feet!'

GARETH: 'I am going to the hospital!'
HEALTHCARE ASSISTANT: 'You ARE in the hospital!'

When the healthcare assistant reaches his bedside, her attention is powerfully focused on completing the morning timetabled task of making his bed. As she works quickly and efficiently to strip and change the sheets on his bed, she does not talk or appear to recognise or acknowledge him or his emotional distress. His frustration is now visible in his body, he sits rigid in the chair, his arms are now tightly folded across his chest:

At 8.10 a.m. the healthcare assistant wheels the large red mobile laundry bag across to Gareth's bedside. She gets things from the 'disposables cupboard' and then wheels the metal trolley piled up with sheets and towels into the bay and starts to strip Gareth's bed.

GARETH: 'I want to go to the hospital or home!'

He looks very unhappy and repeats that he wants to go home a number of times. He is sitting rigid in the chair and now has his arms folded. He does not look happy.

As the healthcare assistant works on changing the bed she says hello to other patients in the bay as they start to stir: 'Morning!', 'How are you?', 'Tired?', 'Breakfast soon', 'Breakfast in a minute', 'BREAKFAST!' As she works, Gareth again tries to stand up. He is pushing down, using the arms of his chair to support himself, but he is not strong enough to get to his feet. He is visibly shaking and struggling with the huge effort of this attempt to stand. He keeps trying and using all the strength he has, but remains in his chair. This is clearly extremely frustrating for him. I also think he may feel humiliated as he seems a very proud and proper person.

Although Gareth had initially expressed his frustration very clearly to the team ('I want to go home!'), over the course of this morning round their attention was focussed on fulfilling the inflexible tasks required within this bay to meet the demands of the wider organisation. He refuses to eat breakfast, rejects all approaches for personal care, and then all further timetabled bedside care during this shift. The impact of the invisibility of his needs on his mood could be seen in the increasing signs of underlying frustration and unhappiness, his attempts to stand up, the tightly folded arms across his chest, when he starts to wring his hands, and, most notably, his later shouts for help and calls for the police and doctors. Throughout the morning he continues to make efforts to stand, but was unable to do so, and thus judged by the team not to be at any immediate physical risk. As he becomes increasingly distressed, however, the team switch their focus on responding to and managing his behaviour as a potential source of disruption to the timetabled work of the ward. Their own increasing anxiety is also apparent in these interactions as they start to speak sharply to him ('SIT DOWN!') and to contain him in the chair; his attempts to stand and walk are now a highly visible risk, potentially both to himself (a 'fall') and to the smooth running of their timetable.

Gareth is still trying to push up from the chair and finally manages to stand up and tells the team 'We need to ring the policeman!'

The nurse responds 'There are no policemen', asking him to sit down. She stands next to Gareth as she fills out the chart of the patient in the neighbouring bed. He continues to use the sides of the chair to stand up. He is very quiet, but there is a strong sense of underlying frustration. He looks very angry. He gets up from his chair again and stands unsteadily on his feet.

> NURSE: 'Sit down my darling, please sit down there, no, please.'
> GARETH: 'I want to see a doctor.'
> NURSE: 'They will be round soon.'
> GARETH: 'No they won't.'

The healthcare assistant and the nurse both move towards him and encourage him to sit back down in the chair. He is now clearly very angry. The breakfast trolley arrives and the breakfast lady (the housekeeper) immediately brings him his tea and toast. He has this every morning. She puts it on his bedside trolley and starts buttering it for him. As she does this, she smiles at him and chats to him as she has done every morning this week. However, for the first time, he doesn't touch his buttered toast. He looks very angry and frustrated. This is worrying – every morning I have observed this week he has eaten four slices of well-buttered toast. He always eats his first two slices very quickly and the team in the bay always get him a second plate of two more slices, which he has always eaten. He is clearly not happy and he has not touched his toast or the cup of tea that is on his trolley.

At 10 a.m. it now feels quite calm and quiet in this bay. All the beds have been changed and all the men within this bay have received personal care and are now in fresh hospital pyjamas apart from Gareth (who rejected their offers), who is still sitting in his chair, hands clasped in front of him and looking very unhappy. The nurse asks him again if he wants a wash now and he responds angrily 'NO'. She moves on to write up notes, remarking 'Let me know when you change your mind'.

> At 10.40 Gareth again starts trying to get out of his bedside chair, pushing down on the side arms of his chair. He reaches out and pushes away the trolley that is. in front of him and gets up briefly. He is very unsteady and has to sit back down.
>
> NURSE: 'SIT DOWN!'
>
> He tells her he wants to go home.
> 'We need to get you safe before you go home.'

> He doesn't look happy at all now. He is starting to look very upset and shouts the words 'GO HOME'. He wrings a tissue up in his hands as he sits in the chair.

It is over three hours later, when he became recognised by the team as disruptive to the timetabled work of the ward (his rejection of all personal care). It is then that they finally focus on Gareth, and for the first time ask him why he wants to leave. He shares his fears about money. Throughout their interactions with him their reliance on routines and their replication of familiar phrases are focussed on reorienting him to accept the tasks: 'Are you ready for your wash?' They focus on orienting him the reality of his situation, that he is in hospital, that he is recovering from a fractured hip, and that he cannot go home. They repeat the name of the hospital, and their roles within it. Gareth does not find this reassuring and for the rest of the day responds by rejecting any and all attempts by staff to deliver care to him.

> At 10.55 the healthcare assistant asks 'Are you ready for a wash?'
>
> GARETH: 'I want my Zimmer.'
> HEALTHCARE ASSISTANT: 'Why?'
> GARETH: 'I want to go home.'
>
> At the start of this conversation this healthcare assistant initially talks to Gareth while leaning over him, but she quickly moves to kneel down, looking up and focussing on him. Gareth tells her that he is worried about his bank account at the post office.
>
> HEALTHCARE ASSISTANT: 'You are in hospital, so you won't be able to go today.'
> GARETH: 'No it's not' (a hospital).
>
> The healthcare assistant repeats the name of the hospital.
>
> GARETH: 'No it's not.'
>
> She shows him the embroidered hospital name that she has on her scrubs. Gareth adds that he doesn't want a wash and they agree. She turns to me: 'It's not worth it, I will keep trying when I can' and documents that Gareth has refused care in his notes.
>
> GARETH: 'I WANT MY ZIMMER!'
> HEALTHCARE ASSISTANT: 'Where do you want to go? You're in hospital, you broke your hip.' She crouches down in front of him: 'Your family are coming this afternoon, they came yesterday. You're not ready to go home yet, you aren't strong enough.'
>
> (Site A day 5)

As this morning progressed, the team responded to Gareth with increased rigidity and patterns of compulsive repetition within their interactions at his bedside, key features of the work of these wards during almost every shift. However, as we can see here - these approaches could rapidly generate significant stress and distress amongst patients and staff.

For people living with dementia, their care needs were often embodied and only apparent in subtle signs that could be identified in their body language and changes in behaviour that indicated an underlying need. Common examples of this that we observed included patients looking uncomfortable, displaying potentially defensive body language, or becoming silent and/or withdrawn. We found that these early subtle signs could usually be traced to later patterns of more entrenched distress and resistance to timetabled bedside care. Importantly, for staff, recognising but not feeling able or allowed to respond to these underlying patient needs during the timetabled work of these wards was associated with emotional and physical burnout.

> The healthcare assistant from bay C comes over to the nurses' station and apologises for her 'little nervous breakdown' earlier. The assistant got upset after being with a patient with dementia who was repeatedly attempting to leave her bed. It is clear she was struggling to respond to this patient while trying to complete the patient observations within this bay. She headed to the sluice room, closed the door but was quite clearly crying, visibly upset by having to argue with and restrain a patient.
>
> (Site A day 1)

Competing and clashing timetables of the wards

As we have discussed (within Chapter 2), there were distinct and competing patterns and rhythms within these wards. The work of the nurses and healthcare assistants was always tightly regimented, focused on the performance and recording of a restricted range of care tasks: this included medication (rounds to dispense medications and also diabetes checks for specific patients), personal care (washing, dressing, changing sheets), continence care (typically referred to as 'toileting' and 'pad rounds'), observation rounds (blood pressure, heart rate, temperature), mealtimes (three main meals), hydration (water jugs and hot drink rounds) and the recording practices that went with them. There were many more, some unique to individual sites, such as the routinised completion of consumption charts, or updating digital displays. These rhythms of rounds and recording flourish within these wards.

Throughout each shift, other medical, allied health, and social care professionals, administrative and auxiliary staff, also entered these wards and attended at these bedsides. These external 'teams' all had their own (often-conflicting) timetables, which, in turn, powerfully shaped the timetables of these wards by appearing to require (this was usually not explicit, but something ward staff typically understood as an expectation) specific tasks to be completed prior to their arrival, most typically during the day shift. For example, the importance of completing personal care and bed making before the arrival of breakfast or the medical teams, and finishing observations before auxiliary teams arrived with meals (as we have seen with the personal care finished before the breakfast trolley arrived, above).

Auxiliary staff also had their own timetables, arriving throughout the shift to clean and remove waste and linen, delivering tea and fresh water, obtain menu choices, and to deliver and remove trays of food. The most prominent allied health professionals were the physiotherapy team arriving to assess and carry out rehabilitation with individual patients, with the medical teams attending for the morning round and less frequently across shifts to examine and assess specific patients at the bedside. However, the timetables of the medical teams were always prioritised at the bedside.

These timetables of the ward (and the competing timetables of teams entering the wards) always dominated and took priority over the timetables (or, more accurately, the patterns of daily life) of individual patients. Regardless of diagnosis, sleeping patients were woken up specifically in order to submit to washes, bed changes, to eat meals, take medications, to be 'turned' to prevent pressure ulcers, or for their blood pressure, heart rate, temperature to be taken during observations rounds. There appeared to be few opportunities for flexibility or a focus on the individual person and their needs within these highly structured and restricted timetabled tasks and routines of care within these wards.

This is particularly significant for people living with dementia, who typically retained and needed their own timetables and schedules and could not easily adapt to these highly structured task-based care practices. It was common for people living with dementia to be woken by the arrival of staff at their bedside, who then immediately attempted to start the fast-paced delivery of the assigned timetabled care or task on their bodies. This could take the form of a healthcare assistant arriving at a person's bedside with a trolley of towels and a bowl of water and to simultaneously start the task of personal care while asking for permission to carry it out. The task would already be underway before the person being acted upon had time to recognise or consent to the care work being carried out on them. Due to the powerfully felt requirement on staff to maintain the timetabled pace of care within these wards, and to complete each task and move on quickly to the next bed, such approaches were not uncommon. These strategies meant that a sleeping or unresponsive person living with dementia could be turned to relieve pressure (clearly a clinical routine where the timing is of significance for patient outcomes), have a spoonful of food pushed into their mouth or have a drinking straw placed between closed lips, as in this example with James.

> The healthcare assistant and nurse are discussing the patient's meal. James is lying flat on his bed, his eyes shut, and appears to be asleep. The healthcare assistant says that yesterday he ate some of the soft option meal, so the nurse, who is 'feeding' patients in place of the healthcare assistant today, goes to the lunch trolley, returning with a bowl of soup, a plate of fish in parsley sauce with a side of mashed potato, and a tub of ice cream. The nurse attempts to 'feed' a spoonful of soup to him, but he still has his eyes closed. The healthcare assistant shouts over the bay: 'You have to sit him up' (he was still lying flat in the bed). The nurse then adjusts his position using the motorised bed. The nurse returns to the food, holding a spoonful of soup. She keeps repeating, 'James, open your mouth … James, open your mouth for

> food'. She does not state what the food is, why he needs it, or what type of meal it is. A healthcare assistant from the neighboring bay passes and says to the nurse, 'He won't open his mouth that one'. The nurse turns to James and admonishes him: 'You can't go home if you aren't eating, that's why you are here', then, more sternly, 'James, when I ask my patient to open their mouths I want them to do it! … Come on, open your eyes and mouth.'
>
> (Site A day 12)

In many ways this highlighted the powerful disconnect between what was considered by ward staff to be the everyday routine work of the ward, as all being of equal value and essential for every patient. Of note here is how the team are anxious about completing this timetabled task quickly (he is not the only person who needs support to eat lunch), viewing him simultaneously as having dementia and needing support, but also able to wilfully reject this support by not eating. It also demonstrates what is missing from many of these timetabled interactions, any recognition of the potential for pleasure and enjoyment of the meal.

Importantly, timetabled care at the bedside typically provided the main opportunity for people living with dementia to make other requests for care and support that reflected their own routine and timetable, some of which could be urgent. However, these requests and needs were always secondary to the timetabled round, and could go unrecorded, or be forgotten amongst the other immediate tasks. It was not unusual for a patient living with dementia to request a cup of tea or a trip to the toilet from the team, only for this request to be acknowledged, but then not carried out, as staff moved quickly on to the next bedside and deliver the next routine task within the timetable. This was rarely intentional, but instead a feature of the primacy of timetabled bedside work over other aspects of care. However, as staff felt the pressure to keep to the timetabled order of care, this could have powerful impact on relationships between staff and patients, which can become visible later in the shift.

Ordering, structure, and fragmentation at the bedside

Within all these wards, there was a strong emphasis on completing specific tasks, to the timetable, but also on delivering them in the organisationally mandated order at each bedside. These tasks were almost always carried out in numerical order, following the structure of the layout of beds within each bay (as we have seen earlier in the care of Sophie in Chapter 3). There appeared to be little flexibility in these routines, and staff could quickly seem anxious and flustered when a task could not be completed in the expected order. The ordering of these tasks was so deeply embedded within these ward cultures that staff rarely stopped a task once they reached the bedside and it was underway. If patients resisted this care, although they could and did move on, typically, staff attempted to complete the routine at the bedside, employing strategies which could range from emphasising the essential nature of the care, to verbally admonishing the patient, or physically continuing to carry out the task on the person, in order to complete it. Only once the task was completed would the team move on to the next bedside in turn.

Here the nurse, healthcare assistant, and a member of the medical team were all carrying out routine work at a bedside. For the nurse and healthcare assistant within this bay they had completed personal care and changed the sheets for most of the other patients in this six-bed bay. As we have seen, this is the heavy and labour-intensive work at the start of the day shift, and after working their way around the bay from bed 1, they arrive at the sixth bedside, ready to work, and speak to Victoria, informing her that 'We are going to change you'. Of note here is that Victoria has been crying and calling out to the staff as they have been working at the other besides, but they have not acknowledged this while they have worked their way, in numerical order, around this bay. Once they do reach Victoria's bedside, they still fail to respond to her cries of distress, instead focussing on their completion of the specific task.

NURSE: 'It's OK we are going to change you'. At first, it is not clear if the team have heard the patient tell them that she is wet, it takes a while before they acknowledge this. Both the nurse and the healthcare assistant put plastic aprons and gloves on before approaching the bedside. They are preparing to change the patient, but before they have closed the curtains around her the consultant arrives to see her. This takes precedence, even though the patient is lying in urine-soaked sheets. She is very angry. As she has been lying here, she has repeatedly been trying to take the wet sheets off, then lying back, still under them, exhausted from the effort. She is shaking all over. The consultant is with her

VICTORIA: 'I CAN'T STAY LIKE THIS.'

HEALTHCARE ASSISTANT: 'It's OK, we will change you.'

VICTORIA: 'I WANT TO DIE.'

The consultant then approaches her bedside and leans over her, asking 'Can I examine your tummy?' The consultant continues, totally ignoring what the patient is saying.

(Site E day 2)

The impact of this strategy, of many different people focussed on carrying out specific fragmented care on people's bodies or at their bedside, was that there appeared to be few perceived opportunities for staff (here the ward team and the member of the medical team) to recognise the person in their care or to acknowledge extreme distress. In addition, during this encounter, the member of the medical team, the consultant, claims and is given priority, even over the removal of urine-soaked sheets. This person becomes reduced to their 'tummy', a body part that must be examined first.

Motion, pace, and fear of 'falling behind'

Motion, pace, and speed were notable features that were highly valued within these wards. The constant motion of staff always on the move, never sitting, conveyed busyness, demonstrating the essential and urgent nature of their roles. Nurses jogged across bays to shut off alarms or sprinted across wards to stop a person from leaving the bedside. Junior doctors walked briskly behind consultants, lined up to 'walk and talk' around the senior clinician. Porters and paramedics pushed beds and chairs in an efficient pressurised style along corridors, as healthcare assistants jumped out of their way as they, in turn, dashed to retrieve piles of linen or equipment from store cupboards and to head behind privacy curtains or into sluice rooms.

A general perception within these wards was that bedside care for people living with dementia took up too much time. As a group, people living with dementia took too long to respond to staff requests, and each timetabled task took longer than allocated, requiring care that often did not conform to the timetabled order. Such care, often idiosyncratic to the individual patient, often with reduced mobility or independence, was typically not recognised as part of the 'appropriate tasks' (Roth and Eddy 1967: 40) of the ward team. These tasks were instead often perceived as a patent's 'whims' and to be discouraged. This led to patterns of increasingly rushed interactions, laced with conflict, as nurses prioritised the expedient delivery of the task (and its recording) over the persons' understanding or willingness to acquiesce to it or that ignored other requests. In turn, these approaches would often exacerbate distress and resistance in patients, making each subsequent interaction more complex and fraught. This would create further perceived delays, in response to which staff increased their pace to make up time, which could all lead to highly charged cycles of resistance to care. This conflict with the routines of the ward could become progressively worse throughout a shift. In this example, not being able to complete this timetabled task quickly and move on to the next patient leads this nurse to exclaim (to the person she is delivering care to, but also to the wider bay of patients, staff, and to us) 'It's a pain in the backside', voicing her frustration at falling behind when an 80-year old man with a diagnosis of dementia, continued to spit out the tablets she placed in his mouth. In response, she used a teaspoon to scoop up the pills and to pry open his mouth and tries to push them back into his mouth.

> NURSE: 'Oh you have spat it out! It's me again! It's a pain in the backside, you need to take them!' She uses a plastic teaspoon to push the tablets into his mouth: 'Shall we try one more?' She puts the tablet on a teaspoon again and puts it in his mouth and tries to give him a sip of juice: 'Can you feel it, it's your cup?' His eyes are still closed and he does not respond. She puts it in his mouth: 'A bit higher darling', she guides it up to his mouth and he takes the cup and raises it to his mouth. She sits next to him: 'Have another sip, have you got it? have a sip darling.' She guides the cup to his lips.
>
> (Site B day 4)

The acceleration of the pace of work, the value placed on speed in the delivery of each task, and onto the next bedside, was only possible with the expectation of prompt patient compliance with (what the ward team considered to be) routine tasks. Here, this nurse focussed on repeatedly establishing the authority of who has prescribed this medication (the 'doctor' and the 'psychiatrist') and her explanations of why Felicity, who is living with dementia, must take the newly prescribed tablet. It is only when Felicity demonstrates, in a number of ways, that she will not take it by disposing of it in her teacup, followed by 'No', that this nurse gives up. She is clearly frustrated and writes this up in the bedside records, but predicts to the wider ward that she will be criticised later for not completing this.

> The nurse goes over to Felicity, taking her medication in a small paper pot. She has a loud voice and a determined pace, which is very strident and stands over Felicity, a tiny elegant woman wearing beautifully coordinated lounge wear, 'I have one little tablet from the doctors who saw you today'. She presses the tablet [Lorazepam] into the palm of Felicity's hand, who in turn closely examines it, and replies: 'It's not the blue one!' She picks the tablet up and straight away drops it into her cup of tea. The nurse's reaction shows she is clearly exasperated with Felicity, 'Look, can I explain to you! Because you have been seen by the psychiatrist today he has given you this.' Felicity is very clear that she does not want the tablet 'No. It's rubbish.' The nurse is now visibly frustrated 'But he has prescribed it … (sigh) OK you don't want to take it?' She puts the rest of the patient's medication away, locking it into her personal drug cabinet: 'It's the first one that has been prescribed!', the nurse mutters, her frustration obvious. She writes in her bedside notes and says to me 'They will say [I] haven't tried!'
>
> (Site E day 8)

This strategy of remaining at the bedside to complete the assigned task was a typical feature of the timetables; however, it often resulted in a further tightening of the schedule with staff using a limited range of (verbal and physical) techniques and approaches to ensure their efficiency, which, in turn, often prompted increasing entrenchment and resistance by the person (as we will also see with Harry in the next chapter). Ward staff often appeared concerned about the consequences of refusal of timetabled care, fearing not only for the patient's well-being but also for their own accountability.

It was rare for a member of the ward team to accept a delay or act of resistance to timetabled care. Instead it was perceived as a temporary nuisance, a feature of the delivery and organisation (the person not awake or just woken up) of the round, to be overcome before moving on, or something to return to later. The institutional demands of the ward routines meant that this was a common experience that caused huge anxiety for nurses, who felt that a task within the timetable must be completed before they could move on to another task or bedside, and that any failure could have significant consequences for them. The medication round was a key timetable that appeared to encapsulate both the practical (the importance for patients to take their prescribed medications) and the emblematic significance (nurses often wore tabards emphasising 'do not disturb' during medication rounds, although, of course, this is of clinical significance) of completing the timetabled task at the bedside. Nurses carrying out the medication round, as in the examples above, would typically appear to feel that they were unable to delay the medication or return to the bedside later, because this was typically a fixed point around which the medications were required to be taken (of course, timing can be critical for some medications) and the wider timetables of the shift could be monitored and stabilised.

Observation rounds were interpreted by ward staff as an essential feature of the organisation and timetable of the ward shifts and these measurements (blood pressure, temperature, oxygen saturation, and heart rate) must be completed and recorded within the patient bedside records (typically secured to the end rail of the bed). However, the observation round and specifically the blood pressure monitor cuff, which was fixed to the upper arm, seemed to cause huge amounts of distress for people living with dementia. On almost every round we would hear patients groan, cry out, and even scream during the inflation of the cuff. However, any distress in response to the inflated cuff on their arm was typically recognised as a feature of their dementia rather than a potential physical impact of the cuff itself (many people living with dementia and older people also has very fragile and easily bruised skin), which was rarely acknowledged. When faced with such responses, although in some cases staff moved on to return later, staff typically continued to attempt to take a recording. As with the medication round (although less common), the observation round typically stalled at the bedside of a patient who found these recording practices distressing. These tasks (taking a prescribed medication and routine monitoring of blood pressure and/or blood sugar) all appeared to have equal significance and value within the timetables.

Timetables shaping cultures of care

Narratives of busyness were deeply embedded within these ward cultures and the professional identity of these teams, and was a regular topic across shifts and during breaks. A focus on the swift delivery of tasks as a means of emphasising the essential and urgent nature of this work emerges. The pace and speed of work was visible in the ways staff moved within these wards, but also reflected their focus. The pace meant that staff often focussed on and identified features of the patient population that might slow these processes, which meant they were less able to see individual people living with dementia or their specific needs or vulnerabilities. Value was placed on the prompt completion of a routine timetabled task, rather than the interactions with patients (or missed opportunities to do so) around them. Stopping to talk to a patient, to listen, or to reassure them, despite its value for patients, staff, and the wider work of the shift (their future cooperation with future routines), was typically overlooked and unrecognised. These interactions could not be quantified or recorded within the available mechanisms, lacked organisational value, whereas the timing and completion of task-based care would be highly visible and documented.

Thus, not only do the patients become secondary to the timetables, but some routines took primacy over others, further relegating the person living with dementia as the least important component in the ordering of these wards. A person living with dementia would be woken up for mealtimes, but this could be interrupted for the competing timetables of medication or observation rounds, while the rounds of the medical team would always take primacy over whatever bedside care was being carried out (as we have seen in the care of Victoria earlier). At the most extreme, we witnessed medical teams give a diagnosis to a woman living with dementia while she was sitting on a commode, and here,

Philip, a man living with dementia, is woken in order to encourage him to immediately eat a hot meal, only to be interrupted for catheterisation, a timetabled task, performed in the middle of his lunch.

> The lunch trolley has arrived. The healthcare assistant and a member of housekeeping begin to serve food within this bay. Philip in bed 1 has his brought out first and he is woken, helped into a sitting position (the team adjust the bed), setting out his hot lunch on the trolley and placing it over the bed for him. As Philip starts to eat the stew, a nurse interrupts and says he can't have it yet. He needs to be catheterised first and that it will only take about five minutes to do. Philip now looks terrified, his eyes darting around unsure and anxious about what is happening as he is partially curtained by the mealtime team. The nurse says to him that he will 'just pop the catheter in and then you can have some lunch'. Philip grunts loudly as he is catheterised. When he is, as the nurse loudly announces, 'All done!', the curtains are opened and the trolley of food is repositioned over him and they present him with a plate of stew. Philip now seems shocked by this experience and looks scared of spilling anything, and fearful of doing something 'wrong'. He is now not eating any of it, he is just staring at the plate of stew.
>
> (Site D day 6)

These disruptions at the bedside, the awakenings, the competing tasks and timetables, reflect what is everyday, mundane, and ordinary for staff, but often strange, extraordinary, and sometimes shocking, for the person, the patent living with dementia in the bed. There also seemed to be very different norms within these wards, with staff accustomed to seeing patients living with dementia 'wetting the bed' or soiling themselves. This resulted in patients' calls for the toilet, or for help following an 'accident', not being recognised as significant or urgent for the person, particularly if staff were already involved with another timetabled task. For ward staff, these were everyday ordinary events, simply a minor event to be expected in the day, another thing to be cleaned up. For patients living with dementia these events could be extremely distressing, hugely embarrassing, demeaning, and powerfully felt.

Conforming to requirements of etiquette and a neat and tidy ward

The timetabled nature of these wards prioritised speed and expedience, but also the completion of tasks in acceptable ways. Tasks must not only be completed on time, but also completed appropriately. This added to the work of these wards and the expectations of behaviour and discipline from the patients under their care. Patients were expected to conform to the requirements of the ward, taking medications, submitting to observations, and eating meals, to the set regiments of the institution, but also to do so in the correct manner. For patients living with dementia, this could be difficult. Eating, drinking, and taking medications are all acts that involve not only swallowing but also eye-hand co-ordination, made harder by being confined within a hospital bed. However, doing so incorrectly, spilling, dribbling, or creating a mess at the bedside was not acceptable here. Yet all of these phenomena are both common and relatively innocuous impacts associated with the condition in its later stages (Archibald 2006). Within these wards, these features instead become deviant. Submitting to the tasks of the ward, but doing so incorrectly, was particularly problematic because any mess or disarray was always highly visible within these wards, where neatness and tidiness was highly regarded as a mark of an organised ward. Furthermore, these relatively innocuous features of living with dementia become highlighted and exacerbated within the person, being viewed as disturbing the ward and creating more work for these teams.

The prioritisation of acceptability in the completion of the timetables within these wards was most prominent at mealtimes. During mealtimes, it was frequently not enough for people living with dementia to eat as and when the ward timetables required, but also to do so in the correct manner. This meant an emphasis placed on eating a meal in order, from the first course (typically soup), followed by the main meal, to the dessert, and to do so in the correct way, sitting up in bed or in a bedside chair, eating from a tray on a mobile table pulled over their lap. Mealtimes could become a key point of conflict within the timetabled routines of the ward as staff emphasised the ward requirements to maintain the correct order and routine of mealtimes against the needs, abilities, and preferences of the person. This could go beyond whether the person living with dementia was or was not able to eat a meal, or requires assistance with it, to staff asserting control over how they were eating it.

> The healthcare assistant (a one-to-one carer assigned to this patient) is talking very loudly to the patient living with dementia in the side room. 'EAT YOUR BREAKFAST SITTING DOWN, NOT STANDING … EAT YOUR BREAKFAST SITTING DOWN, NOT STANDING' The healthcare assistant stands over the patient as he is sits on the bed and repeats this. The patient is wearing pale green hospital pyjamas with a beige jumper with a large logo on the front, over the top of them. His pyjama bottoms are far too long and are puddling around his feet on the floor. He is staring ahead, unfocussed, with a very far away expression on his face. Despite being unresponsive to the healthcare assistant, he has managed to butter his own toast, and has eaten a bit of this and also quite a bit of a bowl of Rice Krispies. The healthcare assistant is now sitting in a chair at his door and whenever the patient starts to stand the healthcare assistant also stands, shouting 'EAT YOUR BREAKFAST SITTING DOWN, NOT STANDING'.
>
> (Site B day 2)

This exchange demonstrates the ways in which staff could begin to exert control over people living with dementia. This is in contrast to many other patient groups, typically younger and of working age, who enjoyed extensive 'privileges' around meals and food choices. They were able to subvert this timetable and leave the ward to obtain food from the hospital cafes or shopping mall, which was something people living with dementia were not allowed to do. There was no medical reason why this man must sit or stand, but it was enough for the healthcare assistant to repeatedly reinforce the order of the ward. Perceived failures to eat 'correctly' caused frustration and could become flashpoints of anxiety for both patients and staff. This could extend to relatively minor aspects of eating, such as using the wrong implement, using a spoon instead of a fork, drinking directly from a jug or flask, improperly cutting up or failing to cut up food, eating with fingers or eating food directly from the tray or table rather than a plate.

The expectations of tidiness and cleanliness are embedded deeply within the routines of these wards. Ward priorities of cleanliness and order move beyond the hygienic and cosmetic, to include expectations that everyday self-care by people living with dementia such as eating and drinking must fit within the established everyday timetables of the ward itself. The need for expedient delivery of care and the maintenance of the timetable can contribute to patients living with dementia being viewed as not belonging, creating mess, and disrupting the ward order. This can be seen here, where Julia, a person living with dementia, is admonished for creating a mess that is a direct result not of her (re)actions, but of the speed at which the healthcare assistant is attempting to 'feed' her:

> The healthcare assistant assigned to the bay approaches Julia, telling the nurse 'I am going to feed her [Julia]'. The healthcare assistant sits down in the chair next to the patient's bed and begins 'feeding' her in a very efficient and functional manner, quickly shovelling full spoons of soup into her mouth. 'NAUGHTY!' She loudly exclaims 'You are getting it all over you!' The soup has spilled onto the sheets, although this seems to be as a result of the large mouthfuls that the healthcare assistant is shovelling into her mouth quickly one after another. 'Open up!', the healthcare assistant says again and again.
>
> (Site D day 11)

To maintain this order, practices often overshadowed the recognition of the person themselves and reduce their opportunities for independence. Julia, the patient above, was never asked if she could or wanted to try to eat independently. A patient could demonstrate independence and a willingness to conform to the timetables of the ward by eating unaided at the set times of the ward, but if their actions, through the impacts of either their acute condition (or their diagnosis of dementia) or that of the equipment around them (eating while lying in bed), created 'mess', it was interpreted as destabilising the order of the ward and such independence would later be denied.

Restoring and tightening of the timetables

Restoring and repairing the timetables was a key feature of the work of these ward teams during almost every shift. Although shifts always started in a determined and orderly way, as they progressed routine care would often take longer than the perceived timetable allowed. It was usual for the timetable of these wards to start 'falling behind' and to appear to break down, and although it was a regular and expected feature of the timetables, it always caused significant anxiety for the ward team. In response, staff (typically during the second half of a shift) typically switched their focus onto repair work, in order to attempt to maintain and restore the timetable. This was characterised by increased pace, rigidity, and patterns of compulsive repetition, at the bedside, which were key patterns in the work of these wards during almost every shift.

The work of maintaining and restoring the timetables was characterised by the tightening of these tasks, reducing them to the repetition of their essential elements at the bedside. As ward staff felt the timetable slipping or escaping them, they increased their pace, and became more rigid in their application. As a result, the needs of patients that fell outside of these essential timetabled tasks, and their restricted remits, became increasingly invisible to them. It was usual for nursing staff to appear frustrated at the length of time it would take to deliver a specific care task at the bedside and in response try to further limit and curb the interactions with the patient at the bedside, to increase the pace, and to move on.

The timetabled routine of the medication round provides a good example of these patterns of tightening. The medication round involved a member of the nursing team dispensing, delivering, and recording each patient's medication, and for people living with dementia (we did not see this approach used with other patients), a process of verifying that the medication had not only been taken but had also been swallowed ('Open your mouth'). This was always viewed as a task that should be a short interaction, a fast-paced straightforward task (embedded within a primary routine of checking and recording the task and dosage in the patient's bedside records) within the overall staff routine and the ward's organisational timetable. This was rarely the case.

The medication round was fraught with myriad potential triggers for fear, anxiety and distrust in the person living with dementia and correspondingly high levels of stress and anxiety for nurses. Unfamiliar staff, unfamiliar medications (even standard medications would often be different in look or dosage within an admission), and fear of side effects (particularly nausea or constipation) were all common (and reasonable) reasons for patients to either question or reject these medications. For nurses, this meant spending considerable time at the bedside, requiring significant explanation and reassurance in order to complete this round of care; however, this complexity and the additional time required was never acknowledged.

In the example below, Sarah is suspicious of the medication that she has been prescribed during her admission. Sarah has a diagnosis of dementia, and her fear of these medications affects not only the nurse, but also the medical team. When the patient cannot be convinced to take her medicine via repetition, coercion is employed by the medical team, the implicit threat being that she will not be able to go home without the medicine. The patient's fear that the medicine will make her nauseous is rebutted but not addressed:

> Sarah is undergoing observation from the nurse, who is quickly able to take her blood pressure and monitor her blood sugar. Sarah seems happy and understanding of this, but is then very suspicious of her new medications.

> The medical team are on the bay, reviewing the patient in bed 9, the bed opposite Sarah. The nurse approaches them and tells the consultant that Sarah is not taking her medication. The consultant goes over to her and says, 'You are clearly desperate to go home, aren't you?' Sarah agrees, to which the consultant responds, 'You need to take your medicine to get home as quickly as you can … the nurse has kindly brought your medicines back.' Sarah tells the doctor that the tablets make her sick. The consultant explains to her that part of the reason she is in hospital is that she is not taking her tablets at home. He then asks her to open her mouth for 'the white one'. He does not give the tablet a name or explain its purpose; she still refuses, and the doctors step back as a group to discuss what to do next, inaudible over background noise of the ward. The consultant goes back and tells Sarah it is Wednesday today and that she can probably go home on Friday if she takes this medicine. He then asks Sarah if she knows why she is in hospital. Sounding rather irate and put out by this, Sarah responds that she feels fine and that she wants to go home. Sarah clearly states that she has two carers at home who can look after her. The medical team again retreat and then return to Sarah's bedside once more. One of the junior doctors suggests she could go home on Thursday. They leave and the nurse, who has stayed throughout, asks Sarah if she is going to 'behave' for her now. The consultant is now conferring with the junior doctors, telling them that it is common for patients obsessed with going home to refuse the medication they need to go home, and that this is a vicious cycle. He describes this as an unavoidable but regrettable feature of the patient's condition.
>
> (Site D day 12)

The work of maintaining and restoring the timetables was characterised by the tightening of these tasks and their rigid application, with the wider needs of patients becoming increasingly invisible to the staff caught within them.

Breakdown and strategies of reactive care

If the tightening of the timetables failed to restore the order of the work of these wards, the timetables could break down altogether and bedside care could become increasingly reactive. As staff felt the timetables breaking down, they typically began to reject the order of delivery and instead start to respond in the moment, prioritising only patient needs that they perceived as 'urgent' or a high 'risk'. This represents an extreme situation for a ward team, and their anxiety in the face of this breakdown of the timetables was very apparent during these shifts. These increasingly reactive responses to patients were strategies to hold back further contagion until handover to the next team.

Importantly, these reactive approaches focussed on care needs that were instantly observable, particularly in response to patient's bedside buzzers, shouting, and calling out, or leaving or attempting to leave the bedside. These patterns of increasing pace, urgency, and reactive care could escalate quickly, impacting on individual patients, but they could also become contagious. The increased tightening of focus, the repetition of aspects of the timetables, and an accelerated pace of bedside care, were all likely to generate significant stress and distress amongst everyone (patients and staff) within these wards, which could spread across cohorts of patients and within teams, and transfer between patients and staff at the bedside. This could have significant impacts on people living with dementia. The increasing noise of patients shouting for attention, additional demands from patient buzzers and alarms, raised staff voices, all, in turn, impacted on a wider group.

Ward teams were then faced with decisions that must be made in the moment, of which patients' personal, immediate, and urgent needs could be deprioritised. Staff were frequently called away from a patient's bedside by other members of their team in response to urgent care needs, as well as by other teams across the ward. The increased atmosphere of urgency generated by the tightening of these timetables often led to staff interrupting each other, and thus either missing or misinterpreting patient needs, with the original purpose of care, and any development of the patient's needs, becoming lost. Multiple members of staff would enter a ward bay and move an object or person, only to leave and have another actor misinterpret the situation and start other types of care.

For example, a healthcare assistant may be supporting a patient living with dementia with their lunch, but be interrupted and leave to help with scheduled care on another bay. At the same time the medical team arrive and push the bedside trolley with the patient's food on it away from the bed so that they can draw the curtains. A passing auxiliary sees the tray of food and removes it to regain a tidy ward. Importantly, people living with dementia, who are typically limited to their bed or bedside, need support with more than just essential care during their admission. When the medical team leaves, the patient living with dementia begins to shout for food, but this can quickly be viewed as irrational to the nurse returning to their bedside, a behavioural feature of their dementia, rather than a rational and reasonable response to the loss of lunch, the invisibility of their needs, and the pace of competing timetables within the ward.

Staff were keenly aware that there were patterns of breakdown and reactive repair work throughout their shifts. Staff knew that on their ward '*It goes in waves*' (site B day 3), or that it is 'always around feeding' (site A day 2), or 'worse around evenings', at the moment when people realise they are not going home and will be staying for one more night (site C day 12). However, staff were typically not able to recognise the potential triggers for these patterns within their wards. Phrases like 'sundowning' normalised these patterns as expected features of a person's dementia, a natural occurrence at a set time of the day; this overlooked the potential impacts of timetabled bedside care, and the ways in which these ward environments created such phenomena. The evening is when visitors are expected to leave, and when patients are left alone. It is the time they become aware that they will not be going home that day. It is the time when the timetables require people to sleep, regardless of need, when the lights are switched off, and when unfamiliar people arrive at the bedside in the dark, such as the next nursing team, arriving for the night shift.

Discussion: The timetables on the ward

Within this chapter we have focussed on the timetables within the daily shifts of these wards, to explore the task-based cycles of bedside care practices, which we found amplified both the behavioural responses from people living with dementia in rejecting them and informed the 'tightening' of the timetabled care practices by staff in response. These cycles of care, and their consequences, supported and reinforced staff beliefs about the recognition and attribution of dementia in the person, and the appropriateness of the application of the diagnosis for individual patients. This category of patient, in turn, became associated with narrow definitions of appropriate care and expectations for the future.

Roth also observed that challenging the timetable of the ward may make a patient visible to clinicians and expedite their treatment, but it also risks going too far, becoming recognised as 'aggression', to which the key response was the reinforcement of the wider timetables of the ward. While Roth observed such phenomena within the larger long-term setting of the rehabilitation clinic, similar responses could be seen within these wards. Even on the wards we observed with the fastest turnover, a patient that pushed the timetables could find themselves quickly transferred or discharged, their personal timetable advanced, but pushed too far, find themselves trapped in a longer organisational timetable of further assessment and monitoring, leading to longer admissions or even permanent institutionalisation (1963: 71). This reflects our observations of the impacts of the timetables of care on people living with dementia in these wards, 60 years later.

Within these contemporary wards, a challenge to the timetable could draw attention to the patient, and could prioritise them for discharge or transfer. However, it could also be viewed as a sign of diminished capacity, behaviour recognised as aggression, violence, refusal of care, which could be understood as the impacts of dementia, but also as a wilful disregard for the timetables of care. For individuals living with dementia, the consequences could be significant. As we have seen with Gareth and Sarah in this chapter, refusal to engage with the timetables of these wards meant a longer admission, increasing the patient's personal timetable and, in turn, their risk of further interventions. Worse, we can see examples such as Mary in the previous chapter, or Claire in Chapter 2, where their response to timetabled care reduced opportunities to go back to their home. Their repeated requests and attempts to go home, typically in response to the imposition of timetables of the ward, contributed to their prolonged admission and decisions about their subsequent institutionalisation within long-term care.

6 Bedside talk and communicating the 'rules' of the ward

Introduction

This chapter explores the strategies and approaches staff used and relied on at the bedside in the care of people living with dementia. Across these wards, we found the rehearsal and duplication of remarkably stable patterns of interactional performance during the routines of bedside care, particularly for this patient group. Of course, it is not unexpected that interactions during the fast-paced work of these wards features well-rehearsed and repeated scripts; however, we found these scripts to be particularly restrictive in the care of people living with dementia. As we have described, people living with dementia do not easily fit within the organisation and delivery of timetabled care within these hospital wards. In response, rather than an adaption to support this significant patient group, we observed increased prescription and rigidity, with talk at the bedside often characterised by compulsive repetition during bedside care for this patient group. Across these encounters, ward staff appeared to pay less attention to the potential needs of the individual in that moment, and focussed on communicating and reinforcing the organisational imperatives: the rules of the ward.

When communicating with people living with dementia, ward staff typically used simplified language and contracted speech, reduced to the use and repetition of key phrases and single words. This typically relied on a handful of phrases, repeated across these wards and sites, that focused on reminding the person of their situation, such as 'You're in the hospital', or simple instructions to be obeyed, 'Sit down!', 'Wait there' and the more blunt 'NO!', which we heard again and again within these wards. This reflected all groups of staff (including nurses, healthcare assistants, allied health professionals, and the medical and auxiliary teams) who typically relied on a restricted, fragmented, and repetitive range of talk. Importantly, these approaches also indicated, to us, to people living with dementia, and the wider ward, staff understanding of 'dementia' as a condition. That the often-compulsive repetition and/or slow annunciation of single words and phrases would aid comprehension, which, in turn, shaped these ward cultures by demonstrating the status of people living with dementia and how to communicate with them *here*.

Of course, all patients are expected to learn the 'rules' of these institutions (Stanton and Schwartz 1954; Coser 1962), 'to learn, and in some way conform to, the rules, restrictions, and freedoms of the hospital' (Stanton and Schwartz 1954: 170). However, although these rules applied to all, we found their explicit reinforcement and emphasis (and an associated emphasis on timetabled care, as discussed in the previous chapter, and increases in restrictions, which we discuss in the next chapter) in the repertoires of communication to people living with dementia within these wards. There appeared to be little potential for flexibility to react to the individual living with dementia and their needs, with a limited range of patient responses viewed as acceptable and in accordance with these organisational rules.

Much of the work carried out at the bedsides of people living with dementia was carried out in silence. When talk did occur, staff repertoires and strategies when caring for this patient population typically opened with the presentation of instructions to be followed and obeyed. Staff often emphasised the potential imminent danger and risks associated with any resistance to these instructions (and the care associated with it). These approaches typically contained a powerful sense of urgency that often displayed the underlying anxieties of the ward team in 'falling behind', as we discussed in the previous chapter. There were frequent appeals to the necessity and expectations of the institution. These appeals emphasised that there was little choice for either the person or the ward team caring for them: '*We have to change you*'. Other tactics we observed, and will discuss in this chapter, included bargaining and the use of incentives.

If a person living with dementia did not respond to interactions at the bedside in ways that were judged as timely and appropriate, it could be perceived as highly problematic for these ward teams. This further underlined the perception that people living with dementia, or a particular patient, did not fit within the remit of that ward. This extended to include any perceived delays in patient responses to bedside talk, questions, or instructions. It became apparent that people living with dementia, who typically needed longer to communicate their needs (both verbally and non-verbally), were often viewed as being both unable and unwilling to comply. This perceived unacceptability could take many forms, including difficulties in communication, and any behaviour viewed by staff as resistance to care, disruptive, or inappropriate, or when patients expressed other additional urgent care needs. This could also extend to include people living with dementia making clear statements requesting further details about their care (such as medication or treatment changes) or declining care. Patients living with dementia were typically given few opportunities to question or interrupt care as it was delivered to them. Ward teams often appeared not to recognise or acknowledge a patient saying 'No'. As in the case of Sarah (see Chapter 5), rather than acknowledging these acts of agency, saying 'No' was recognised as a feature of a person's dementia, an inability to understand the context and rationale of the care offered to them. In others, as in the case of James (also Chapter 5), this could also be interpreted as a 'wilful' rejection of the ward rules. This further reinforced understandings about the condition, its recognition in individuals, and the commonly accepted notion amongst staff that this group of patients did not belong on their wards.

We observed that the 'medication round' was a key point within the everyday timetables of bedside care, where these patterns of communication and their consequences could be prominently observed. During the dispensing of bedside medication, the majority of encounters with patients were unproblematic. However, when examined across whole bays and wards, it was rare for this timetabled care within a bay of four to six patients to be completed without any perceived delays. Instead it was typical for this routine to stall at numerous bedsides, particularly within bays where people living with dementia were commonly cohorted together. Across these wards and hospital sites, we observed that the interactional performance and routines of the medication rounds varied little. At the patient's bedside, we observed different nurses (only nurses can administer medications within these wards) duplicating specific phrases and interactions (with their consequences also being reproduced) during medication encounters with the same patient living with dementia across a shift, but also over the days and weeks of an individual's admission. Importantly, we found these scripts to be particularly restrictive in the care of people living with dementia, where these approaches often accelerated into patterns of increasingly repetitive talk and of conflicts that could result in the patient's behaviour being understood as a feature of their dementia, while at other points they were also viewed as wilfully disruptive to the work of the ward.

We observed the care of Harry for 15 of the 20 days of his admission within a Trauma and Orthopaedic ward. He is 100 years old, does not have a formal diagnosis of dementia (however, he was often described by ward staff as having dementia) and had been admitted with a hip fracture, a '*left hemi*'[1] and was five days post-operation at the beginning of our observations. At handover that shift he was described as having '*abnormal*' urine, and that '*he was very wheezy yesterday*'; it was queried whether he had 'hospital acquired pneumonia'. He also had profound hearing and sight impairments. Harry had spent his entire admission confined to his hospital bed (across wards this was described as being 'bed bound').

Throughout his three-week admission, the routine medication rounds became a routine and established flashpoint of conflict and struggle between Harry and the nursing staff. Each time, Harry would methodically ask for more information, asking for more details of the medications they were giving him, explanations of what they were, and questioning what he was being asked to take and why. These medications did not match those taken in his usual routine at home. The tablets were different shapes and sizes and there were more of them. However, Harry's questions were always dismissed by the nurse administering the medication as both unnecessary and time-consuming. Over time, their exasperation with his requests became very clear to both Harry and the wider ward. These interactions further underlined and reinforced to staff that he did not fit within the remit of their ward; in response, this led to new labels and classifications being assigned to him. His subsequent decline during his admission became expected and viewed as inevitable.

> Harry is fast asleep, his head is propped up on the pillows and he is covered by a thin sheet, with his bare feet exposed and uncovered. He doesn't move.
>
> The nurse arrives at the bedside and he stirs. The nurse informs him it is time for his medications and this becomes a discussion about his medication, covering what he needs to take and when he takes it:

Harry is very insistent 'I have three tablets for my heart.'

'They have been stopped by the doctor.'

'Have you got them? I have to take three tablets.'

Harry lifts up three fingers for emphasis.

'The doctors have stopped them because of your blood pressure.'

'Have you got them?'

'Yes, they are here.'

'Why can't I have them now, straight away?'

'Because of your blood pressure, it's too low, OK?'

'But I can't see the point of it!'

'Now I am going to do your eye drops.'

The nurse begins to lean over Harry in preparation.

'Just a minute!', exclaims Harry, stopping her.

'It is taking me half an hour to explain it to you!', says the nurse. She is clearly starting to get exasperated. 'Can I do your eye drops?'

'I want the capsules for my heart.'

'You can't.'

'You've given me an eye drop. I need a blood test.'

At this point a healthcare assistant comes over and interrupts the conversation. She begins to talk to Harry, using his first name frequently. The healthcare assistant explains to him: 'The nurse is trying to give you your eye drops. Let her give you your eye drops or it will be late.'

'I haven't had the capsules, I don't want any more eye drops.'

'Listen, the doctor doesn't want you to have them because your blood pressure is too low' The healthcare assistant begins to raises her voice.

'Well how are you going to make it higher then?'

'They are checking you and you will probably have more blood, but we have to listen to the doctors'. Harry seems to respond to this, so the healthcare assistant repeats it. 'We have to wait for the blood results.'

'OK.'

'Do you want your breakfast now?'

'Yes.'

'Here's your Weetabix.'

'Yes, but what about my tablets? I take three tablets for my heart.'

'The doctors don't want you to have that.'

'OK, they said that?'

'Your Weetabix is here.' She places the tray on his lap on the bed and he focuses on eating his Weetabix.

The healthcare assistant and the nurse look worn out by the exchange. They look at each other and laugh gently to each other, before looking over to me.

(Site E day 1)

As we have discussed (within Chapter 5), the medication round within the timetables of these wards was always a time of increased urgency and often increased anxiety for nursing staff, which was driven by perceived organisational constraints of completing this task efficiently and the importance of patients taking all of their (typically multiple) medication(s). Staff expressed a clear sense of relief and accomplishment if this round was completed without perceived delay. However, it was common for people living with dementia to query their medication, either expressing concerns that the medication offered was not the same as their home prescription (including variation in brand, dose or delivery of familiar medications) or apprehension of medication that they feared would have side effects (such as nausea or constipation). Although this was a predictable and everyday feature of these routines, it was always viewed by staff as 'disruptive' and 'challenging', which appeared to increase everyone's anxiety, stress, and frustration.

> 9.30: The Nurse looks exhausted. She is rubbing and stretching her back. We are only two hours into the shift. We chat and I say it is a moment of calm.
>
> 'Don't tempt it!' she retorts, quickly. This is very common, with all ward teams saying 'Don't jinx it!' Calm is viewed as rare and short term. 'They are all fine, but I don't know any of these patients, they are challenging! I don't know how long I was with [Harry], but it seemed like half an hour! But I was running out of things to say. I was glad the healthcare assistant came along! I was on a loop for about half an hour!'
>
> (Site E day 1)

This frustration is also linked to the visibility of the medication round. When a medication round had not been completed, nursing staff appeared to feel exposed to the scrutiny of others in the institution for this apparent failure to complete their task (as we have seen in the previous chapter). However, the team rehearse a limited number of phrases and approaches. Despite Harry clearly stating 'I don't want to take anything, there is uncertainty', the team persist. Across these encounters they become increasingly prescriptive and rigid, with their talk to him at the bedside characterised by compulsive repetition. They repeatedly enrol the rules of the ward, that it is the 'Nurse's job to do the medication' and that 'You are in hospital now'. I observed these interactions as this nurse describes it 'on a loop', repeated by two different nurses on the following day shifts (days seven and eight of his admission) and at no point did staff share information about what reassurance Harry required during the administering of his medications.

> As Harry eats lunch, the student nurse and nurse arrive at his bedside, where they begin to discuss his tablets. Harry looks at them and begins to question the medication again.
>
> 'I don't want to take anything, there is uncertainty. I want my daughter to sort it out for me.'
>
> 'It's the nurse's job to do the medication.'
>
> 'I know that.'
>
> 'We are doing what the doctors say.'
>
> 'I take a capsule.'
>
> 'This is a capsule, once a day.'
>
> 'Can you say the name?'

The nurse says the name of the capsule.

'That's right. That is definitely right.' Harry repeats the name of the drug. The nurse places the tablet in his hand. They discuss the shape of the tablets.

'Three little white ones', the nurse says, as she puts them in his hand.

'That's wrong.'

'Why?'

'They are not my heart tablets.'

'Sometimes tablets come in different shapes and sizes.'

'I know the ones I take it's long.'

'It's a different size but it's the same medicine. You are in hospital now and there are different suppliers, the name of the medicine is the same, the name is the same.'

The nurse keeps a gentle conversational tone of voice at all times. She tells him that she is reading the drug chart for him. Another nurse from a different section joins them at the bedside and repeats that it is the same drug, it is just a different shape.

'Shall we pour them in for you, into your mouth?'

The nurse puts the tablets into his mouth and the student nurse gives him a sip of milk. Harry takes the tablets.

'Sorry for being so awkward', he says.

They note this in the chart and the student then asks if he is ready to take his eye drops. They agree and she talks him through the process, reminding him there are two drops in either eye.

'Are you ready?'

The student nurse lowers the bed so that Harry is leaning back. She puts in the first drops.

'This is a quick process. Two for each eye.'

Harry asks when he takes these.

'Morning and night'

'You've just done that.'

'No. It's two different drops.'

'She leans over him.'

(Site E day 6)

Staff typically employed this restricted script of talk and techniques, without listening to him, and there was little reference to his questions and concerns. Different approaches were used in turn as each failed to obtain the appropriate or required response: the patient's acceptance of their request, to allow the delivery of care to continue, and to comply with the expectations of the ward. Of course, it is unsurprising that staff within these wards followed scripts during these repetitive routines of bedside care. Here, however, any perceived failure to respond to them and meet their requirements, set people living with dementia apart as not belonging.

These patterns of conflicting expectations, between the needs of Harry to understand what medications he is being asked to take and the insistence of the nurses that he comply, and their underlying anxiety at the length of these interactions, was repeated during every medication round. In this instance, it resulted in Harry being reclassified. Harry was recorded as resisting bedside care, with his behaviour viewed as both a feature of his (undiagnosed) dementia, but also as wilfully disruptive. Harry became perceived as a patient who did not meet the requirements of the ward, somebody who did not belong there.

Despite the complications in Harry's condition (he is still confined to the bed and has a chest infection), he is moved to a low-dependency bay. Here the nurses worked at a faster pace at the bedside, had even less tolerance for perceived delays, and expected compliance without question. Their interactions with him at the bedside transformed from a general weariness at his questions into something more clearly dismissive. These approaches also informed others within this bay (as we can see in the reactions of both the medical team and other patients in the bay) about the accepted ways of talking to Harry. The fieldnotes at the time document concerns about the impacts on Harry. He seems 'more diminished and frail' as his admission progressed.

> 9.30am. Harry was moved from the high-dependency dementia bay and has been transferred to the low-dependency bay. The nurse is at his bedside and snaps 'That's what I was doing, you told me off!' Her demeanour is very harsh and firm with him. She sounds frustrated and he seems a bit more diminished and frail. She shouts directly into his right ear [he is deaf in the left ear] and they begin a long discussion about his tablets. This follows the similar pattern as previous conversations about his medications:
>
> 'Here are your tablets.'
>
> 'Which one? Is it the heart one?'
>
> 'Yes.'
>
> 'That's the right one…'[…]
>
> 3:00 p.m. Harry is talking loudly. 'I need a doctor to talk to me, we need to sort this out, I have been waiting seven days.'
>
> A younger man in a neighbouring bed shouts at him: 'SHUT UP, SHUT UP, SHUT UP!'
>
> On the opposite side of Harry's bed a group of medics are with another patient. They clearly hear this exchange, but they do not respond or intervene.
>
> Harry continues, 'I have my ear piece in I need to talk to someone.'
>
> This continues for some time and is quite upsetting to hear. Harry looks very vulnerable and has changed significantly since he was moved from the high-dependency bay.
>
> (Site E day 9)

This new tone continues throughout the further interactions ward staff have with Harry at his bedside. This coincided with a pronounced deterioration in Harry's condition. By the 18th day of his admission, he has an infection and is transferred to a private room. Over his admission, these patterns of interactions appear to inform ward understandings of Harry and his potential for recovery. The team rationalise that this deterioration is an inevitability associated with his age and his dementia. The nurse in charge discusses his case:

> He's got an infection and he got a lot worse and at his age, one hundred, he just can't take it. He's down (in the handover sheet) as 'Do Not Resuscitate' and they have filled out the (DNR or Do Not Resuscitate) form.
>
> (Site E day 13)

I visit Harry again and talk to his daughter and granddaughter who sit holding his hands. They look scared and bewildered at what is happening to him. When I arrive in the ward the next day, I immediately see that there is a new person in the bed. I was expecting this, and I feel a huge sense of sadness, fatigue, and loss. He has gone and there is no trace of him.

Working in silence

The institutional hierarchies and the organisation of these wards also appeared to prevent communication between ward staff and also between staff and people living with dementia. Despite the typically fast pace and busy nature of the work within these wards, and the detailed interactional work involved in care delivery, much work within the ward and at the bedside was often carried out in silence. This could serve to reinforce the invisibility of patients and also some categories of (typically auxiliary) staff. Here the team of cleaners were deep cleaning a bay; they did this work silently, not talking to each other or to the patients as they moved the furniture (including occupied beds and chairs) to clean around and under them. This could be extremely disconcerting for patients, particularly people living with dementia. For example, David, who is living with dementia and is also visually impaired, is lying in bed, could feel his bed being moved. Although he asked what was happening, he obtained no response. Later that morning, we chat and he asked me where he was and I reassured him he is still in the same place. David thought he had been moved to somewhere new, somewhere unfamiliar.

> I go into the bay, it is really noisy because the cleaning team are 'deep cleaning'. This involved moving the beds and furniture into the bay or across into another patient's space, sweeping the floor, using a really noisy floor cleaning machine that uses soapy water (this is disinfectant giving off a strong smell), and then a drying and buffing machine, again very noisy, and then moving the furniture (and the patients) back into place. David is in his bed and is moved by the cleaners. However, they don't say anything to him as they do this. They are always silent and don't speak even when he asks them where he is. When they leave I check on him; he seems quite anxious and thinks he has been moved to a different room
>
> (Site C day 5)

Rigid and repetitive talk

As we discuss in Chapter 5, bedside care was always viewed by staff as essential care. Thus, although staff would acknowledge a patient's immediate concern or need at the bedside, they would quickly work towards reorienting the person to the reality and rules of where they were, what had happened to them, and what must happen to them. We found these patterns of care to be particularly restrictive and impactful for people living with dementia. Although it was usual to seek permission from patients before care was carried out on the body, and staff gave the appearance of seeking permission, the delivery of care was typically already happening or quickly continued regardless of the patient's response. A tacit assumption of assent was always made, with an overriding sense that staff felt they were acting in the person's best interests. Any further talk focussed on obtaining the correct response from the person to allow care, or to continue with care, and generally occurred as staff worked on their body. This was often most overt during what could be seen as the least essential and non-clinical aspects of timetabled bedside care, such as the daily personal care routines early in the morning shift, where the completion of care was typically fast-paced.

Staff approaches at the bedside were highly repetitive and rigid, focussed on emphasising the rules of the ward. Staff typically presented instructions to be followed and obeyed, often emphasising the potential imminent danger of patient actions and these instructions typically contained a powerful sense of urgency that often displayed their own underlying anxiety and fear of delays and 'falling behind'. Appeals to the necessity and expectations of the institution were made routinely, and these emphasised that there was no choice for either the person or the ward team caring for them: '*We have to change you*'. This talk could also include bargaining, with future activities, visits from family, mealtimes, or going home frequently used as incentives. Looking nice for visits, being dressed for a meal, or submitting to interventions, or observations in order to go home, were all commonly used inducements.

These patterns of discussion, negotiation, and bargaining occurred within an incredibly asymmetric power dynamic. These exchanges provide ways of uncovering aspects of the social standing and loss of identity of people living with dementia experienced during an admission. It is important to note how much of this highly repetitive talk was directed at reminding the patient of their place in the world, and the rules that needed to be followed. However, ward staff also emphasised their own status in the ward; they must all fit the expectations and timetables of the institution.

What surprised us was how incredibly constrained and rigid this script was and how consistently key words and phrases were used amongst all staff, including nurses, healthcare assistants, auxiliary, allied health professionals, and medical teams at the bedside of people living with dementia. This extended to their consistent pattern of use across all these hospitals, despite the geographic spread and demographic variance of our sites. This talk was directed at people living with dementia, with very little time given to listening to them or allowing them the opportunities they required to express their needs. Similarly, the repetition of simplified stock phrases or words repeated and enunciated at increasingly louder volumes, and slowly articulated, was frequently deployed as an approach expected to increase patient understanding. Potentially complex requests were reduced to single word abstract statements, such as 'LUNCH?', 'WASH?' or 'TEA?' There was typically a certain institutional tone of voice and also discomfort apparent in much of the bedside talk, as we can see in this encounter when a senior member of the medical team arrives at Daniel's bedside:

> Daniel's eyes are closed and he is talking gently to himself. Throughout his admission he appears to be in a very dreamlike state. His talk is like a gentle stream of consciousness. It suggests he has visions of faraway exotic locations. The nurse and student nurse reach his bedside with his drug chart. 'Hello, my love, I have your painkillers here. What's your date of birth? Can you tell me? Lovely'. She passes him a glass of water.
>
> A senior member of the medical team arrives, asking 'How is he doing?'
>
> 'He is doing OK.'
>
> DANIEL takes a tablet and water.
>
> NURSE: 'One more… (to the medic) he's quite mobile.'
>
> MEDIC: 'Previously he was mobile, but…'
>
> The medic stands over the bedside: 'Hello sir, how are you? How is your walking coming along?'
>
> DANIEL: 'It's coming along… you can't force it… It will continue.' Daniel says this with his eyes closed and in a gentle dreamy faraway voice.
>
> The medic seems quite posh in his tweed jacket. He looks very traditional in his smart country style clothes. He is very tall. He stands in front of Daniel and looms above him. He is high up. He seems quite awkward as he hovers and ends the consultation: 'I like your positivity! Keep trying!'
>
> DANIEL: 'Oh I will… I will'. Again he talks in a dreamy and wistful tone
>
> MEDIC: 'WELL DONE… WELL DONE… I will come and see you tomorrow'.
>
> He strides out of the ward.
>
> (Site A day 8)

In contrast, many people living with dementia, despite these widespread assumptions made about the impacts of their condition, often responded eruditely and knowledgeably. They would often give clear reasons why, for instance, they disliked and preferred not to take certain medications and would give reasonable reasons for interrupting or resisting these forms of bedside care. This ranged from those able to state that a certain type of medication makes them nauseous, that they do not like certain food, that they need to get up to go to the toilet or to wash. They would, however, often receive the same limited response from staff that would be used to people living with dementia across these wards, despite the wide range of individual patients with their own unique needs. Ultimately, the timely delivery of the task, the requirement, for example, to take the medication the pharmacy has sent, to consume the food sent by the kitchen, or to stay in bed, always overrode the wishes of the individual patient.

Talking to people living with dementia about their hospital admission, they described to us the ways in which these limitations were powerfully felt and not being listened to had profound impacts on them. Here, Paul, who lives with dementia, describes the impacts of these approaches, and how it 'knocks your confidence'.

PAUL: Patronising, infantile, like I said that I mightn't be able to hear properly or understand properly and all they had to do was ask instead of making those assumptions. So you do feel very childlike and, you know, it's not good, it's not good, it knocks your confidence completely and no one should be making assumptions about anybody.

(February 2019)

These standardised strategies at the bedside also included the use of the taken-for-granted 'institutional lingo' (Goffman 1961 {1991}: 55); the host of acronyms, job titles, and medical jargon that all patients and their families were expected to understand, alongside familiar words given new meanings, without explanation, within these wards. While the language of these wards was highly stylised, there was an assumption that it was universally understood by all within it. Names of wards, of procedures, and of hospital processes, were routinely used without explanation. This was particularly problematic for people living with dementia, who, despite their mental acuity, physical dependency, and expectations for recovery being constantly queried and subject to scrutiny and assessment, this was often judged through their failure to recognise and respond as expected to the host of potentially unfamiliar acronyms and language of these wards. A patient usually had no prior knowledge that in hospital a 'BM' is a blood glucose monitoring test, yet a person living with dementia will be approached by staff that are 'just doing your BMs my darling' several times a day. Similarly, the regular statement of 'I'm just going to check your pad' followed by an intimate examination (there were routine and regular checks to see if continence pads were 'wet' and needed changing) was assumed to be understood by people living with dementia.

Incongruous phrases were often used, in particular by staff visiting or passing through the wards. A person in a uniform or scrubs would respond to a patient calling them and asking for immediate care or urgent support, by telling them 'I'm not on this ward', 'I don't work here', or 'I'm not on here', without context or explanation, creating unintended distress for these patients. These narrow repertoires of language, the restricted patterns of speech, and the inclusion of the unfamiliar, were most prominent at the bedside, during the delivery of the most mundane aspects of everyday care.

Standardised routines and strategies at the bedside

Staff typically employed a cascade of interactional techniques at the bedside, used, in turn, as each failed to obtain the appropriate or required response: the patient's acceptance of their request, to allow the delivery of care to continue, and compliance with the expectations of the ward. Any perceived failure to meet the requirements, set people living with dementia apart as not belonging within these wards.

Here, the team draw on a well-rehearsed cascade of techniques: they start by asking Kevin if he wants to get out of bed, to which he responds: 'No, leave me here'. They then emphasise the necessity of this, move on to appeal to the requirements of others (the physiotherapy team and his family) and propose making a 'deal'. They move from making what seems like a general enquiry, to emphasising the necessity of their request. It is only at this stage that they reveal the underlying aspect of his care they must complete, they tell him they need him to get up from the bed so that they can check if the continence pad that have put on him earlier needs changing: 'We need to check your pad'. They go on to further emphasise the essential nature of this care: 'we must'. They reinforce the reality of his situation by reminding him of what has happened to him (his broken hip), to finally stating what must and is going to happen: 'We are getting you up'. Throughout this encounter the team discuss together their rationale, emphasise his autonomy and his ability to decide 'I won't force him'. Although this also implies that this may end soon. However, as soon as they reach the bedside, they start to work on Kevin's body as they talk to him. When they complete this task and he is sitting in his bedside chair, they praise him, and reward him with a chocolate; they seem highly relieved that the demands of the organisation have been met.

> Kevin is lying in a bed that is low to the ground. The nursing team go over to him and ask him if he wants to get out of bed.
>
> 'No, leave me here.'
>
> 'Your daughter will be here soon and you were going to walk with the physio for her, you need to be up in the chair when your daughter arrives… your family will be with you soon and they will like to see you up in the chair, are you sure?' (Kevin shakes his head) 'I am not going to force you but it would be good to have you sitting up. Make a deal, we will give you this morning to rest and get you up later in the afternoon. We just need to check your pad.'
>
> 'I am not well...'
>
> 'We still need to check the pad for you.'
>
> The physio brings him a black coffee as she promised. It is in a black ceramic mug. 'A proper cup', she puts it in front of him. He is really grateful and puts the radio back on as promised.
>
> 'Kevin, we must get you up this afternoon… I won't force him, it's not fair, he can still tell you what he wants, it's not fair.'
>
> They draw the curtains back and sort out the bedside around him and tidy up the trolley. There is a lot of chocolate on his trolley and they tidy it up to one side of the surface. They give him some chocolate, and ask 'Do you want some water?' They pass him some water with a straw and he drinks it. The nurse then helps him to open a sweet wrapper.

This exchange was additionally complicated for this patient because their request was actually signalling a requirement, to allow the delivery of essential care; however, he does not recognise this code. Throughout the talk at the bedside, staff used coded language that patients living with dementia were expected to pick up on, understand, and comply with. As was often the case, Kevin did not recognise this and instead reasonably believed they were offering a choice, which results in them starting to view him as a person who does not meet the expectations or rules of the ward. The team quickly return with a hoist and after a similar exchange, they use it to lift him out of bed and into the chair and reward him with another chocolate.

> 'Kevin, there we are, don't you feel better sitting in the chair? For all that hard work would you like a chocolate? I thought that would make you feel better.' She gives him a chocolate from the bowl on his trolley.
>
> 'I wish I could be like you, you've got life in you.' Kevin says this to the patient in the bed opposite.
>
> 'It's been a long struggle though.'
>
> The student nurse says to Kevin: 'He's been in here longer than you, that's why.'
>
> Music plays in the background - '...and the beat goes on ...and the beat goes on...'. contrasting with the harsh bleep from the seat alarm '....the beat goes on....'.
>
> Later they check on Kevin again: 'Are you OK in the chair now?'
>
> 'It wasn't that bad was it, can I do your blood pressure and pop this on your finger?'
>
> (Site C day 6)

The team now quickly move on to take Kevin's blood pressure and other measurements that must be recorded in his bedside records. It is also important to consider the intensity of this detailed interactional work, in terms of the highly repetitive strategies and phrases staff used and switch between at his bedside. These bedside routines were not bundled together, but were separated out into individual timetabled tasks that must be carried out at each bedside in turn, often provided by different members of staff within the team. Thus, these exchanges were repeated again and again throughout a shift as staff moved from bedside to bedside.

The rules of the ward

Across these wards, staff talk to patients living with dementia at the bedside typically addressed the person by locating and reorientating them very clearly in relation to the reality of where they were, what had happened to them, and the expectations of the institution. This reflects a primary understanding of dementia among ward staff as predominantly one of cognitive deficit that requires continual orientation and verbal cues to indicate the reality of their situation. By far the most common, widespread, and indeed almost universal approach staff used at the bedside, was to locate the person as being within the institution: '*You are in hospital'* or, more typically, a loudly enunciated *'YOU. ARE. IN. HOSPITAL!'* Staff would routinely emphasise, to the point of compulsive repetition, the reality of what had happened to the patient living with dementia and why they were there: '*You have broken your hip', 'You have had a fall', 'The doctor is coming to speak to you'*. This talk focussed on reorienting the person to the rules of the ward and signalling accepted behaviour within the context of its routines and timetables.

However, an incredibly common impact of this approach was that it could cause an individual patient living with dementia to become extremely anxious, afraid, unsafe, and fearful of what had happened and where they were. This led to an extremely predictable loop we saw repeated again and again across these wards, staff would quickly declare '*You are in hospital'*, which would trigger anxiety and fear in the person living with dementia. Ward staff would then respond with further repetition, often simplified to 'HOSPITAL', joined by other ward staff, using increasingly loud voices, simplified speech, and repetition, reinforcing this message, as if repetition would produce comprehension. For example, it was not unusual to hear many staff repeat this, as on a loop, to a person living with dementia *'YOU ARE IN HOSPITAL... YOU ARE IN HOSPITAL... YOU ARE IN HOSPITAL..'*. [Site B day 3].

This cycle of increasing rigidity, repetition, and volume of speech was typically applied if the person living with dementia did not appear to respond quickly enough, nor respond in the expected and permitted ways, or if they did not become pacified by these repeated rationalisations. However, these approaches typically amplified anxiety. For many people living with dementia, and older people in general, the thing they feared was the hospital and what their admission might lead to (as we can see in the case of Caroline and Lauren below). By reorienting patients to recognise their place within the hospital, staff inadvertently recreated and reinforced clearly verbalised fears that this admission would lead to institutionalisation, the fear that this time they would not be allowed to go home.

> Caroline is being admitted and is currently sitting in the corridor with a relative. All of the nurses agree she has some cognitive impairment. Her son suspects dementia, which the nurses agree with. She has been attending a memory clinic, but is not yet diagnosed. One nurse tells me she is 90 and 'doing amazing'. The nurse in charge tells me she has refused all care except medications, which are her home prescription. She is aware of the setting, date and year, but very angry. Wants to go home but lives alone. She refuses to be changed (into a fresh continence pad) and reacts angrily to being touched by the team. She is sore (from the soiled continence pad), but won't let the nurses address this. There is a lot of discussion about what to do. The nurses are wondering how they can move her, the Registrar is concerned that it is not safe for her to be on the unit, while her son is concerned that she is a danger to herself anywhere else.
>
> Thirty minutes later, Caroline is back on the ward (via the coffee shop) and is sitting in a wheelchair flanked by family. The healthcare assistant and her son are trying to encourage her to eat. She refused breakfast and they are worried that if she doesn't eat she will get worse. Caroline speaks very

> clearly. She tells the healthcare assistant that if they make her eat she will vomit it. Her son offers to take her home, but the nurse says she can't leave as they want to do a mental capacity check. The registrar is worried that despite her clarity she is not rationalising things 'correctly'. For the next twenty minutes her son continues to encourage her to eat. He is worried she will be in a worse condition later if she does not eat, and the nurse encourages him to continue encouraging her.
>
> I speak to the nurse. She says the anger is understandable. The patient has been able to use coping strategies to disguise cognitive decline up to now, but they can no longer work. However, the doctors will not assess her capacity until she has settled, so by refusing care she is managing to put off any assessment and diagnosis.
>
> Ten minutes later, a doctor approaches asks Caroline if she can remember what they are monitoring. Caroline gets angry at this. She questions why people are questioning her memory and says she has had enough. She goes from calm to angry to defensive, making the memory test impossible. The doctor, a physician associate, is unflappable. She reassures her, she agrees with her, she maintains a clear and calm tone. The patient's daughter then starts talking to the doctor, so the healthcare assistant begins to talk to Caroline, who gets angry at having to keep repeating herself to different people.
>
> Thirty minutes later, the nurses go over to Caroline again. She is initially calm but becomes angry when asked if she can remember the fall (the cause of her admission). Says she won't say again and starts to complain about her son. She is extremely wary and defensive of their questions about her memory and won't have it discussed. If she is asked a question twice she quips back: 'You have already asked me that and forgotten but no one is asking you questions. My choice if I go home to die, it's my life.'
>
> (Site E day 2)

Typically, staff ignored or directly contradicted these immediate concerns and during these encounters, ward staff appeared to be actively trying to support and help orient the patient to the reality of where they were and what was happening. However, this approach always appeared to increase the person's anxieties and fears and triggered further resistance and rejection of care, such as in this case.

In this next example the team either only briefly acknowledged or did not respond to the anxieties that the patient, Lauren, expressed throughout their encounter at the bedside. Lauren is clear in her anxieties. She wants to go home, she is worried about the cost of her hospital admission, and she wants to know where her family are. While all of these issues are reasonable concerns, they are quickly dismissed. For staff, these questions are familiar irritants to be ignored, while for patients living with dementia such as Lauren they are an expression of real and immediate concerns and anxiety. The team respond by repeatedly and compulsively reminding her of where she is, 'You are in hospital', as though being repeatedly informed by strangers leaning over her bed would be reassuring and a panacea to her anxiety. It is also of note here that the healthcare assistant and the physiotherapist, despite having very different roles and training, have virtually identical scripts.

'Lauren, do you want to go to bed?' Asks the healthcare assistant.

'NO! I want to go home!'

'You are in hospital, you are in hospital.'

'I can't afford it.'

'It's free.'

Lauren rubs her arm where the bandaged IV port sits, and begins to run her hand along the long tubing, which leads up to the mobile stand that supports her IV drip.

'It's for your medicine.'

'I don't like being here. I don't know it.'

'I know, you are in hospital.'

Lauren takes the orange juice pot left over from her from lunch, puts it into the sip cup, and places it in front of her on the tray table.

'Where is my son?'

'He will be here soon.'

The physiotherapy team arrive on the bay and come over to Lauren's bedside. The pair are very young and sporty, dressed in matching polo shirts embroidered with the hospital logo.

'Hello, Lauren.'

One physiotherapist stands next to Lauren while the other goes to fetch a walking frame from the bed opposite.

'I am NOT staying here!'

One of the physiotherapists crouches down beside Lauren and looks up at her.

'At the moment you are in hospital… you are in hospital.'

Lauren continues to look agitated.

'Look around. There are other patients in here. You have hurt your hip.'

'Where is my son?'

'I am sure he is coming later. Would you like your cardigan?'

Lauren has been sitting wearing just her pink hospital gown and now they have mentioned it she does look cold. They get her cardigan from the cabinet and help her to put it on she instantly looks more comfortable.

The physio then asks her: 'What country are we in?'

'I don't know. I can't afford to pay for it anyway.'

The physio decide to give up and to leave her. They move on to another patient.

(Site E day 4)

At the end of this encounter, the physiotherapist suddenly adds a question that appears to be assessing Lauren's cognitive capacity, 'What country are we in?', but which also comes across as jarring and out of context. Its incompatibility with the natural and expected pattern of this conversation could constitute a form of scrutiny that is additionally disorienting and stressful to her. Here we can see the ways in which a person's failure to be pacified and reassured by these repetitive statements could become recognised as a feature of their dementia and interpreted very quickly as a potential sign of cognitive deficit.

These informal assessments or 'memory check' questions occurred frequently during bedside care and exist outside of the standard cognitive tests, as discussed earlier within Chapter 3. These questions were often enrolled by staff, particularly when the patient was not meeting the organisational expectations and rules of these wards; in turn, however, they could also further disorient them. They feature as an extension of the assumption that the linguistic reinforcement of being 'IN THE HOSPITAL' should be enough to simultaneously reassure any patient of their anxieties and remind them of the behavioural norms of the institution.

Many of these exchanges revolved around a patient expressing anxiety about their admission, such as concerns about the length of their admission and wanting to go home, or reasonable and rational questions and concerns about the rules of the institution. Patients worried about how to pay for aspects of their care, including meals, clothing, slippers and toiletries, as they would elsewhere. Such fears would often be viewed in a light-hearted way by staff who appeared amused and dismissive. More often, they would respond with an answer that only made sense with a understanding of the setting or its economy, 'Don't worry, you are in hospital' or 'It's the NHS'. In the case below, a patient is worried he is not able to pay for his care:

> According to the handover notes, Simon, in bed one, appears to have some form of cognitive impairment, if not dementia. He stops a member of the medical team and asks if he has to pay for treatment, he sounds very worried. He repeats that he is not sure if he can afford it. She tries to reassure him, saying 'It's the NHS', before continuing with her rounds.
>
> (Site B day 14)

This extended to visiting family, who also typically reminded the person of the reality of their situation, often repeating the common phrase 'You're in hospital' [site C day 3]. However, for families, this could also extend to reminding the person of what has happened to them and also their family, as here, reminding Kevin that his wife had died recently. This highlighted the difficulties and discomfort for families when the person appeared suddenly unable to remember key events or people, potentially reflecting a sudden change in their cognition, with family responses typically focussed on reorientation, reminding the person, and willing them to recall recent events and the reality of their current situation both in and outside of the hospital.

> Kevin's middle-aged daughter has been sitting with him and as she passes him chocolates, she has been listing all of his friends who have died before him, emphasising that he the last in his group of friends to survive. 'Mum's not here anymore remember?' She gets up and leans over and kisses him: 'See you tomorrow'. She leaves the ward. Kevin's wife died three months ago and he routinely asks for her and looks for her in the other beds in the room throughout his stay and this continues after she leaves.
>
> (Site C day 5)

The use of these reorientation approaches is actively discouraged in much of the literature within long-term care, which instead encourages staff to engage with the person's reality as much as they can. In the acute setting, however, the needs of the institution, the importance of recognising the rules of the ward to enable the timetabled routines of care, overrode this, and patients' realities were routinely challenged, even though we found that this routinely caused anxiety, and fear in people living with dementia.

Instructions for following the rules of the ward

Staff focussed on providing instructions to people living with dementia, which typically contained a powerful sense of urgency that often displayed the underlying anxiety and fear of staff within these wards. During these exchanges, staff often raised their voices as they gave very clear and often-simplified instructions to the person living with dementia, '*SIT IN THE CHAIR, SIT DOWN*' [Site B day 3], often giving these instructions standing at the foot of their bed or standing over the person.

These rationalisations also typically included repeated warnings emphasising the potential risks, imminent danger, and the likely consequences of their behaviour if they did not comply and failed to modify their behaviour. Of particular concern for staff was the risk of people living with dementia 'falling' or 'having a fall'. The example below is typical of interactions heard all day, every day, within these wards, as staff repeatedly instructed patients to stay in bed, or to stay sitting down, or they will fall.

> 'Get back into bed.'
> 'NO!'
> 'You will end up falling.'
> 'NO! NO!'
> 'You will end up falling.'
> 'Get into bed. It is night time.'
> 'NO!'
> 'Are you staying in bed?'
> 'NO!'
> 'What will happen if you fall?
> 'If you were a doctor you would help me.'
> 'If you fall you will be in hospital longer.'
> A patient in another bed shouts across the bay 'You are an idiot!'
> 'You can go home if you are better, so please stay in bed.'
> The healthcare assistant stays with him for a while.
> 'Put your leg back in. You will fall.'
> 'I didn't fall once.'
> 'They asked me to stay here because you have fallen.'
> 'GET OFF!'

The healthcare assistant stands over the patient, watching him as he twitches his legs on the bed.

(Site A day 18)

This also demonstrates the ways in which a patient emphasising their wishes was viewed as particularly problematic and repetitive behaviour, and became the focus of concern for staff, who, in turn, responded with highly repetitive approaches. In the example above, this patient's repeated attempts to get out of bed becomes an urgent focus of staff control. Importantly, this becomes recognised as both a feature of his dementia, but also a wilfulness and rejection of the rules of the ward, which overlooked other potential underlying need, and no one asks why he wants to leave the bedside. The perceived immediate risk of 'falling' overrides any potential for a person having rational agency. It also reflects the prioritisation of the needs of the ward, for which the monitoring of 'falls' are a key marker of care quality, over the needs of the individual patient. This further demonstrates the ways in which ward staff perceive these patients as not belonging within these wards. The behaviour of people living with dementia are reduced to a risk to be managed to meet the rules of these wards.

All are required to meet the rules of the ward

Appeals to the expectations and requirements of the institution was commonly used to persuade people living with dementia to accept care, and this typically emphasised that there was no choice for either the staff members or the person: '*We have to change you*'. In this case, the healthcare assistant initially asks the nurse in the bay to help her to change the wet soiled sheets. She emphasises to the patient, Ted, who is living with dementia, 'We need to move you' and 'We can't leave you' while he remains lying in bed (fractured hip). Ted is now shouting '999', the number for the emergency services, which indicated his fear about what is happening to him and that he believed he was being attacked in his bed. The shouting alerts the wider team and several healthcare assistants join them behind the curtain, providing additional help as they struggle behind the curtain.

The nurse and healthcare assistant are back at Ted's bedside. 'Sorry Ted.'

The staff keep using the shortened version of his name, but also keep forgetting whether his name is Ted or Edward.

'GET OUT! GET OUT!' He shouts at them.

The nurse responds first to the healthcare assistant, then to Ted:

'He is soaking we are going to have to change his sheets… You are wet.'

She asks for more help and asks a healthcare assistant in the team in the next bay to help them to roll him. She goes back and says to him: 'We need to move you… it's not good to lie in a wet bed.'

In response, Ted shouts '999!'

'We are just going to change the sheet.'

'YOU CAN LEAVE ME ANYWHERE YOU LIKE!'

> 'Come on now. We can't leave you in here.'
>
> The healthcare assistant from the other team comes into the bay, sanitises with hand foam and then puts gloves on before she goes behind the curtains to help.
>
> 'Right Ted, you need a new sheet.'
>
> He is clearly struggling with them behind the curtain and is clearly not happy. His moans and groans can be heard from outside of the curtain. They draw back the curtains. Ted looks very very frail. His head is resting on large white pillows. He has been left wearing a blue hospital gown, with a sheet and a thin blue blanket neatly and tightly tucked in around him. The side bars on either side of his bed have been pulled up.
>
> (Site A day 4)

Once care was completed, the patient is safely contained within the bed (the side bars have been raised); however, we do not know the longer-term impacts of this on the person. Ted appeared to believe he was being attacked and in response more staff appear at his bedside. His response was viewed as a feature of his dementia, but the number of people surrounding him and carrying out intimate care, changing his continence pad, cleaning him, and changing his clothes and the bed sheets, causes distress in the moment, but the potential longer-term impacts on Ted are not considered here.

Discussion

Although this chapter has focussed on interaction and 'talk' within these wards, it must be noted that ward staff rarely spent significant time with individual patients living with dementia, and during our time within these wards, it was rare to see a member of the ward team feel they were able to take time to sit with, listen to, and have a conversation with, a patient living with dementia. Overwhelmingly, these ward cultures discouraged and frowned upon staff sitting or even pausing in their work, with 'sitting' only permissible while working on the body or updating patient records (we will discuss this in more detail within Chapter 8). Encounters between ward staff and patients living with dementia occurred predominantly during the fast-paced delivery of care on the patient's body at the bedside, or when in motion 'while they were 'on the move' and with head averted, or no response at all' (Rosenhan 1973: 255).

This talk typically emphasised the traditional 'Doctor's orders' (Coser 1962: 73), whether this was to emphasise the importance of completing timetabled care or to dismiss a patient's immediate concerns or requests that could potentially derail the delivery of care. This suggests that the interactional work with people living with dementia at the bedside has not kept pace with ongoing and significant developments in understandings of patient consent, capacity, and decision-making. It is important to note how much of this talk took place as staff were already working on the patient's body, reminding the patient of their status and the status of ward staff caring for them, reinforcing the need to learn and conform to the rules of the institution.

The organisational approaches within these wards emphasised the task-based and repetitive nature of bedside care, which meant that these incidents of care work were understood as straightforward transactions. There was little recognition of the complex reality of these 'tasks' or the potential for variation in individual need (Menzies Lyth 1959). There was a pervasive sense that because the organisational structures divide bedside work into tasks, this assumed the interactional work should also be straightforward and routine from patient to patient, thus taking a standard Fordist-type amount of time for each task within the wider timetables of the shift. This denies the complexity of caring for people living with dementia, which requires sensitive and nuanced interactional skills, particularly of listening and the recognition of embodied communication, which requires a slower pace. Yet these were skills that were neither recognised nor valued by these institutional cultures, which emphasised pace, urgency, and the requirement to deliver care in a particular format, to a set order, and at a set time. The raising of the side bars at the end of the interactions with Ted in the example above were quite typical. In this we can draw parallels with Butler's work on linguistics. Butler (1997) argues that the performative nature of speech can take away power from people and groups, creating vulnerability and precariousness as it does so. In many ways, this is what we found within these wards.

These patterns of interaction and the language of these wards that we have presented in this chapter were the same across roles and professions, from ward staff, medical teams, allied health professionals, and auxiliary staff. We found that the language and interactional approaches, the specific phrases they used at the bedside, also lacked distinctiveness that reflected a recognition that these were encounters with individuals. They appeared standardised and interchangeable, often reduced to simple phrases or single word commands to the point that ward staff often did not appear to recognise when their speech deviated from expected norms, appeared strange or incongruous, and could make little sense to the person living with dementia (or indeed any person) in the context of the specific situation. Yet such approaches could be heard being endlessly repeated and rehearsed in the bays and corridors of these wards across these sites. Because the language of these institutions was so embedded in these wards, there appeared to be an expectation that this must also be comprehensible by all. This gives an insight into understandings of dementia as both a cognitive loss, one that could be remedied with constant and compulsive repetition of contracted phrases, and where failure to respond as required by the organisational mandates could simultaneously be recognised as a feature of a person's dementia, but also viewed by staff as a wilful disregard for the rules of the ward.

Note

1 This is an intracapsular fracture which requires a hemi-arthroplasty (half-hip replacement) which involves removal and replacement of the ball of the hip joint.

7 Organisational cultures of containment, restriction and restraint

Introduction

Within all of these wards, we identified that a significant feature of the organisation and delivery of care for people living with dementia was the use of containment, restriction, and restraint. These approaches to care were typically embedded within these wards' organisational cultures as a response to the behaviours (resistance to timetabled care, and behaviour viewed as disruptive, inappropriate, or transgressive) of people living with dementia who were viewed by staff as 'challenging'. We suggest these practices could be more widespread, constituting the everyday bedside care for people living with dementia during a hospital admission. Importantly, these approaches were not applied to other patient groups, and the restraint of people living with dementia within these wards was both a response to such 'behaviour', but, in turn, also frequently generated resistance and further patient distress. We now explore the ways in which the organisational mandates and drivers informed these everyday and taken-for-granted cultures of restraint and their impacts.

The use of restraint in the care of people living with dementia is, of course, governed by complex legal regimes; however, when we refer to its use within these wards, we are not talking about the commonly imagined form of physically tying down a patient. Instead we refer to practices that go beyond the legally recognised or the easily quantifiable, to the limitations and restrictions placed on the 'privileges' and freedom of people living with dementia during an admission, particularly on their movement and mobility.

We observed a wide range of practices that were part of the everyday cultures of routine care within these wards. Beyond the use of highly restrictive language (as we have already discussed in Chapter 6), we observed several everyday approaches and techniques to restrain patients which were never questioned in their application within these wards. These included the raising of the bedside rails or bars, and tucking bedsheets in tightly around the person in order to contain and restrict a person living with dementia within their bed. For those sitting at the bedside, furniture such as the mobile tray table would be placed close to the patient to restrict movement and the ability to stand, with technology to encourage movement, such as walking frames, placed out of reach. Technologies such as chair alarms not only restrained people to their bedside chairs, but also alerted staff to any attempt to breach this containment. Clinical technologies, including continence technologies (particularly the routine use of continence pads, bed pans, and commodes at the bedside in the care of people living with dementia), and tightly secured medical equipment, also limited movement from the bed and bedside. These were routine practices typically embedded within the organisation and delivery of everyday bedside care.

Other everyday practises of restraint included 'specialing'. Returning to the specialist language referred to in the previous chapter, the hospital ward is one of the few places where the term 'special' is used as a verb rather than an adjective. Individual patients and even whole bays were 'specialed', while staff were also described as 'specialing' a patient. In reality, this meant little more than assigning a member of staff, typically an agency worker, a healthcare assistant, or student nurse, to provide direct supervision to a patient or patients. 'Specialing', and the use of alarms attached to chairs and beds, had been explicitly introduced and categorised as 'safety measures' by these institutions with the goal of reducing risk and improving the care of people living with dementia. In reality, they often appeared to be little more than institutionalised forms of containment and restriction, principally employed to minimise the number of falls recorded on each wards.

For us, restraint was a feature of care that we never imagined, and the frequency in which it was used took us by surprise. It was not at all in our sights when we entered these wards, nor something that we were actively looking for. However, it was powerfully present in our fieldnotes from the very first day within these wards. This use of restraint had significant consequences for people living with dementia, and also for the staff caring for them, shaping and transforming the cultures of care within these wards.

These practices reflected institutional and clinical priorities and were principally informed by the goal of improving patient safety, to prevent injury to the patient (falls and fractures), and to minimise risk (ensuring they receive essential care) to people living with dementia, and these aims were typically vocalised by staff during bedside care within these wards. Safety, reducing risk, and, specifically, the risk of further injury, of 'falls', 'wandering' or 'absconding' during an admission, were significant concerns embedded in the organisational drivers within these wards; recorded falls has become a key metric in measuring ward performance and care quality. However, across all these sites, these organisational concerns had become transformed within these wards into cultures that prioritised keeping the person living with dementia contained, restricted, and restrained, within their bed or sitting at the bedside. Staff expressed high levels of concern and anxiety about all people living with dementia in their care leaving the bed or bedside, and this increased exponentially if they were walking in the bay, the wider ward and corridor, or moving towards the ward exit.

We know, from wider research, that a focus on safety can prevent serious injury and harm. However, these widely used practices had other powerful and largely unacknowledged impacts on these ward cultures, shaping the priorities and pace of work, which had detrimental impacts on both individual patients and staff within these wards. It could also reduce opportunities for people living with dementia to regain mobility and independence, cause significant patient distress and anxiety, and of emotional distress and physical burnout for ward staff.

Importantly, although these practices of containment, restriction, and restraint, at the bedside were tools for achieving patient safety, meeting the institutional priorities and performance metrics, and maintaining the organisational demands of the timetabled order of these wards, they also frequently triggered the very phenomena recognised as those features of dementia perceived to require restraint (resistance to timetabled care, and behaviour viewed as disruptive, inappropriate, or transgressive), further categorising the patient living with dementia as not belonging, as 'challenging', and thus requiring restrictive intervention.

We found that these phenomena of institutional 'looping' (Goffman [1961] 1991: 41) were widespread, in that the practices of tightening the timetables, the work of communicating the rules of the ward, and the use of containment and restraint at the bedside, generated the very behaviours staff recognised as dementia that required these care practices and interventions. As Stanton and Schwartz (1954) identified, we too found that many of the routines and procedures reflecting the organisational priorities of these wards, contributed significantly to these patterns of behaviour in their patient population: 'As our recognition of such sources of continuing conflict became clearer, we began to wonder if staff procedure and attitudes contributed to and helped maintain chronic patterns of behaviour amongst patients and staff members' (1954: vi). To the use of restraint in response to disruptive behaviour triggered by the admission (Jones et al. 2006). We also wondered if these patterns could be more closely associated with and to the cascade of decline, known as cascade iatrogenesis (Thornlow et al. 2009).

Intensification, contagion, and 'collective disturbance'

Importantly, these approaches to containment, restriction, and restraint constituted part of the tightening of the timetables (within Chapter 5) and the compulsive communication of the 'rules of the ward' (within Chapter 6) we have described earlier in the care of people living with dementia, and which manifest, as Menzies Lyth identified within the hospital wards she spent time within in the 1950s, through the 'increased prescription and rigidity and by reiteration of the familiar. As far as one could gather, the greater the anxiety, the greater the need for such reassurance in rather compulsive repetition' (Menzies Lyth 1959: 63). These patterns were visible to us in these contemporary wards, in the reiteration and widespread enforcement of the practices of containment at the bedside, which seemed to be applied automatically and viewed as part of necessary everyday care at the bedside for people living with dementia.

A patient living with dementia leaving their bedside or walking within these wards was overwhelmingly categorised by ward staff as a high-risk and deviant action. In response, ward staff typically utilised a range of strategies, as we see here, in the care of Camille below, to limit the person within the bed or at the bedside. This usually involved repeated efforts, featuring highly restrictive and repetitive talk and containment practices that included shadowing a person living with dementia as they walked, barring their way, and attempts to encourage or instruct the person to return to their bedside. Any apparent resistance to these efforts typically increased and heightened the levels of restriction experienced by the person living with dementia. However, this strategy typically generated further resistance and increased the person's distress and fear about their situation. It also meant that their underlying or urgent needs often remained unexplored, unidentified, and unmet, or significantly delayed. However, these patterns also had consequences for ward staff and contributed to their experiences of stress and anxiety during these shifts.

Here, Camille, who is living with dementia and was medically fit to leave, was simply waiting for her 'package of care' (as discussed earlier in Chapter 3) before she can return to the care home in which she was living, is walking away from her bedside. The healthcare assistant gives her a walking frame to use but immediately uses this to change the direction in which Camille is heading, leading her back to the bedside. This restriction makes Camille very angry and her frustration is clear to all. In response, the healthcare assistant reminds Camille that she cannot leave her; she does not comply, however, continuing to walk out of the bay, and trying to open the doors at the end of the ward (which leads to storage). At this time the healthcare assistant takes the frame from her and turns it around to face into the bay. During this encounter, this healthcare assistant emphasises the expectations of the ward for both of them: 'I can't leave you alone', repeatedly reminding her of the rules of this ward. 'You need to go back to bed' and eventually resorts to instructions to be obeyed 'turn around'. However, by the end of this encounter Camille is very tearful, shaken, and afraid. She begins to shout in frustration, vocalising a desire to be left alone. This encounter increases attention from other staff within the ward, who begin to crowd around her and repeat the earlier instructions, further intensifying her restriction and amplifying her fears and frustration. Eventually a different member of staff joins them, suggests a cup of tea, puts an arm round her, and leads her back to her bedside:

> Camille has just woken up, gets up from the bed and walks slowly away from the bedside. The healthcare assistant gives Camille a walking frame to use (she has taken this from another bedside), stays with her and turns the frame to lead her back to the bedside.
>
> Camille shouts, 'LEAVE ME ALONE!' She is very angry and wants to keep walking away from her bedside.
>
> 'I can't leave you alone… hold onto it [the walking frame] with both hands.'
>
> Camille heads back to her chair, the healthcare assistant stays with her, but then turns around and, using the frame, keeps walking out of the bay and into the ward corridor. The healthcare assistant stays with her, shadowing her closely, just a step behind, with her arms crossed. Camille turns to her sharply:
>
> 'LEAVE ME ALONE!'
>
> 'I can't leave you alone.'
>
> Camille continues walking up and down the corridor using the walking frame until she arrives at the double doors at the end of the bay. She looks through the glass panels of the doors and tries to open them (they are not locked but no one uses these doors and they don't lead anywhere other than to a storage area with broken equipment). The healthcare assistant immediately

steps in, stops her and asks her to turn the frame around and to go back. When this doesn't happen, the healthcare assistant takes the frame from Camille and turns it around to face into the ward. Camille is now shaking with rage. 'LEAVE ME ALONE… I WISH YOU WOULD LEAVE ME ALONE!' she screams, her frustration and rage palpable. This leads to increased attention from other staff within the ward who head over, crowd around her and repeat the instructions to return to her bedside. One of the physiotherapists goes over to her; she is very smiley and warm. She says 'Hello' and puts an arm around Camille, leading her off down the corridor:

'I wish she [the healthcare assistant] would stop following me around! I am not going anywhere!'

Camille is very angry and frustrated. They walk back down the corridor and stop by one patient's bed to say 'Hello'. 'Have you been good?' Camille then walks along the corridor to the end of the bay with the physiotherapist, before turning around and coming back again. All the nurses, healthcare assistants, the hostess and the cleaners that she passes all talk to her. They then return to the bedside where Camille sits down. The healthcare assistant brings her a cup of tea.

'I'M FINE JUST LEAVE ME ALONE!'

A little later, Camille again uses the frame to walk into the corridor. Again, the healthcare assistant shadows her and tells her' 'You need to go back to your bedside'.

'DON'T TELL ME WHAT TO DO! NO ONE CAN TELL ME WHAT TO DO!'

'Well you need to go back to bed.'

The healthcare assistant follows Camille as she reaches the corridor and tries to leave through the double doors at the end of the bay. The healthcare assistant now tries to turn Camille around by steering the frame around, along with the clear instruction: 'No.'

'LEAVE ME ALONE! GET YOUR HANDS OFF ME!'

'Turn around.'

Camille is really angry, incandescent, but also seems very afraid and upset: 'Yes have a good laugh! Leave me alone. leave me alone.'

The physiotherapist sees this and comes over again. She smiles at Camille and says, in a very bright and cheery voice, 'Hello Camille! Come with me!' She puts an arm around her and steers her down the corridor in the other direction.

'I don't like her [the healthcare assistant]. She's too bossy.'

Camille looks very upset now, on the verge of tears.

'How about a nice cup of tea?'

The physiotherapist puts an arm round Camille's shoulders.

'The nice cup of tea is waiting for you over there.'

The physiotherapist points to the trolley next to Camille's bed. She leads her back to there and helps her to sit down.

'There's a nice cup of tea there.'

> I chat afterwards with the team.
> 'It doesn't always work!', says the physiotherapist.
> 'It all kicks off sometimes!', responds the healthcare assistant.
> (Site E day 2)

There appeared to be no immediate risk to Camille in walking within this ward (she was classified as 'self-mobilising') and it could benefit her rehabilitation (and relieve boredom) prior to discharge. Yet for the ward staff these patterns of repetition and intensification in their use of verbal and physical containment and restraint were part of the everyday work of this ward. There were, however, powerful impacts on patients like Camille and the staff caring for them during these encounters. They generated distressing emotions for Camille, the very phenomena recognised by the ward team as requiring restraint (resistance to timetabled care, and behaviour viewed as disruptive, inappropriate, or transgressive), further categorising her as a 'challenging' patient, and thus requiring restrictive intervention.

We also observed powerful patterns of contagion; once one person living with dementia in a bay or ward became distressed, particularly if they were shouting or screaming, this could have powerful impacts on other people (particularly other people living with dementia) in the bay and the wider ward who could become fearful and distressed. It also further intensified the restriction practices of staff in managing a larger group of distressed patients while also maintaining the timetables of care. Camille's distress and her struggle with the team powerfully impacted on the other five women living with dementia within this bay. In turn, when they became distressed (particularly one woman who routinely screamed out in pain when the blood pressure cuff was applied during the observation rounds, and another who had hypoactive delirium), this would also impact on Camille, increasing her fear of the ward and prompting her attempts to leave the bay.

These patterns of looping and contagion were a regular feature of the shifts within these wards and appeared to be a form of 'collective disturbance' recognised within much earlier ethnographic accounts of life within hospital wards (Coser 1962; Stanton and Schwartz 1954) where a 'mood sweeps in the general atmosphere… the majority of patients on a ward become upset at one time' (Coser 1962: 88), which could also lead to 'sporadic outbreaks of violence and anxiety' (Stanton and Schwartz 1954: 392) and 'contagion' (1954: 395), where 'the disturbance had spread to include many patients and personnel' (1954: 386). These patterns have a long history as a phenomenon recognised within institutional life (1954: 294), which have traditionally reflected long-term institutional populations, occurring over considerable periods of time. However, within these contemporary wards, this was typically a phenomenon that occurred routinely, and in some wards daily, most likely to occur in the afternoons or at the end of the day shift and the start of the evening shift. Importantly, although many people living with dementia clearly expressed their distress at these restrictions, for many, this distress and anxiety could also manifest as extreme withdrawal.

As these patterns, cycles, or loops, of containment and escalation manifest during a shift, ward staff could also appear to increasingly interpret their role as one of management and containment, associating all movement by people with dementia as a significant risk that should be minimised and controlled. We too found this constituted part of the tightening of the timetables and repetition of practices, which has a longer history, and identified by Menzies Lyth within acute hospital wards in the 1950s (Menzies Lyth 1959: 63).

An ordinary and taken-for-granted aspect of ward cultures

The use of restraint in the care of older people (and other vulnerable populations), of course, has a longer history and encompasses a wider range of practices across sites of care. However, its contemporary use in the care of people living with dementia has received relatively little recognition or attention. People living with dementia are at significant risk of experiencing containment, restriction, and restraint during an acute hospital admission and are more likely to be restrained than any other patient group (DeSantis et al. 1997; Minnick et al. 2006; Gerace et al. 2013), with reports of recorded restraint over ten times higher than for patients admitted without dementia (DeSantis et al. 1997).

Restrictive practices for this hospital population does not take the commonly assumed form of physically tying down the patient, although the use (internationally) of what would be commonly recognised as restraints (for example, vest, waist, and wrist restraints) continues to be reported (Evans et al. 2003; Hynninen et al. 2015; Muñiz et al. 2016). Instead, in the hospital setting, contemporary practices of containment, restriction, and restraint go beyond these quantifiable methods and instead encompass a wider range of taken-for-granted practices that are embedded within the everyday cultures of care.

Within this chapter, we refer to a wide range of measures used during routine care, often viewed within nursing cultures as a 'necessary evil' (Griffiths 2013). The many limitations placed on the freedom of people living with dementia during an admission, particularly their mobility, typically with the goal of ensuring patient safety (Hughes 2008), to prevent injury to the patient (falls and fractures), to minimise risk (ensuring they receive essential care), and as a protective practice (Coleman 1993), carried out by staff across hospital systems. Internationally, forms or restraint are recognised as often poorly documented, undocumented (Kirkevold and Engedal 2004; Evans et al. 2003; Meyer et al. 2009) and covert (e.g. the use of tray tables) (O'Connor et al. 2004). This reflects the widespread use of 'indirect approaches', such as keeping people undressed, removing walking aids, the placement of equipment, and verbal commands not to move (Saarnio and Isola 2009; Lejman et al. 2013; O'Connor et al. 2004; Liukkonen and Laitinen 1994; Muñiz et al. 2016), or interventions recategorised (as in the case of chair alarms, and one-to-one care within these wards) as 'safety measures' and 'positional aids' (Minnick et al. 2007).

The restraint of people living with dementia appears to be deeply embedded within the organisational cultures of ward care. Its use reflects the ward priorities and the challenges of maintaining the timetabled, task-list systems of care (as we have seen within Chapters 5 and 6) (Moyle et al. 2010; Natan et al. 2010; Houghton et al. 2016), viewed by staff as the 'shortest route to compliance'

(Borbasi et al. 2006: 306), to ensure the wider work of the ward can continue (Wang and Moyle 2005). Staff described using restraint to manage people who were considered to be 'out of control' (Moyle et al. 2010), when they 'bother others', or when their clinical needs or behaviour is believed to require more intensive forms of support (Hughes 2008).

While there was some variance in their application and frequency, the multiple repertoires of containment, restriction, and restraint, we identify within this chapter were ordinary and common practice within all these wards. For example, the practice of containment within the bed was so unexceptional, that people living with dementia were described by ward staff as '*climbers'*. The everyday, ordinary, and commonplace technique of raising the side rails of the bed may have originally been designed to prevent people from falling, but had transformed into a method of containing people within it; of tucking bedsheets in tightly around the patient; adjusting the motorised bed into unusual positions (e.g. raising the patient's feet, or both head and feet); all restricted and confined people living with dementia within their bed. For those patients sitting at the bedside, the tight placement of the mobile tray table close to the body pinned the person in place; walking frames and wheelchairs were placed out of reach at the foot of the bed; alarms attached to bedside chairs and one-to-one care were all used as containment practices. All of these actions were automatic, routine, ordinary, deeply embedded, practices within everyday cultures of care, tacitly understood as necessary and required approaches for the care of people living with dementia within these wards, rather than a considered reflection of the needs of individuals within it.

We found that the use of everyday items within these wards to support these practices was not limited to the bed and bedside chair. Almost all routine clinical technologies within these wards had a dual use when applied to the person living with dementia. The most common example of these were continence technologies. We found that the routine use of continence pads and, especially for men, catheters, along with bedpans and commodes, appeared adapted as a means to keep the person living with dementia contained at the bedside. The use of continence technology effectively minimised and reduced the need for the patient to leave the bedside, further legitimising the restriction of movement. Other everyday technologies applied to the body primarily for treatment and care (e.g. bandages) were often used in ways that reinforced the requirements to remain at the bedside.

We did observe infrequent and limited use of chemical forms of restraint (medication to inhibit behaviour or movement). We cannot, however, make any claims about the underlying reasons for its use, nor its dosage, as we had only limited access to patient medical records.

Ward life experienced as incarceration

Many patients living with dementia described their experience of ward life as a form of incarceration. Even a short stay of a few days could be highly distressing for people living with dementia, and within these acute wards, many experienced admissions lasting many weeks, even months. Although they had typically recovered from their admitting condition and were subsequently classified as 'medically fit to leave', people living with dementia were often not 'permitted' by their multidisciplinary team (the 'MDT') to leave and return home (or return to long-term community care) until an assessment and any requirements for social care support had been put in place. All of this led to delays in which a patient with no medical condition must stay contained and restricted to the hospital bedside.

As we have described (within Chapter 2), these wards typically had little stimuli, with many having limited access to, or no TVs, radios, or newspapers. They were boring, and when they were not boring, they could be frightening. Should the person living with dementia attempt to leave the bedside, to overcome boredom, or due to fear of their surroundings, during this time, then they could quickly become classified as resisting care, their behaviour viewed as deviant, disruptive, or inappropriate, and forms of restraint applied.

This had powerful impacts on patients and here, Patrick, who is living with dementia, repeatedly tells us that he feels '*like a prisoner*'. He has remained in his bed and bedside chair in this bay for the two weeks of his admission. His has been concerned about his things and has often been worried about where his things are being placed, particularly his electric shaver. He tells me that today he is very worried that he will not be able to watch the racing because he cannot operate the pay-per-view television screen at his bedside. He describes his frustration at the ward and the staff. He does not understand why '*They [the staff] take things away and they don't bring them back*'. He cannot make sense of the rules of this ward.

> Patrick is sitting in the bedside chair. He is wearing hospital pale green pyjamas and red hospital issue socks. The mobile bedside trolley is in front of him with a small glass (with an inch of water in it) a big bag of chocolates and the Sunday papers (his niece had visited him earlier). When he wakes up I go over and say hello and ask him how he is.
>
> 'I am very frustrated and angry, it's like being in a prison here, one minute they say keep drinking and then next they won't let you… [he is on a restricted fluid intake] …No one tells you anything in here, this is like being a prisoner! I want to watch the racing tomorrow. I am very worried that I will miss it. I can't work this thing or put any money on it, I can't work this thing… [he points to the TV]… it's Tuesday, Wednesday and Thursday, it's important to watch it'. I reassure him that I am in tomorrow and will remind the team and make sure it is working.
>
> Later on, he says to the man sitting opposite: 'This is terrible we are never going to get well like this, it's like being in prison… (He looks very fed up)… They take things away and don't bring them back.'
>
> (Site C day 9)

More often, though, the distress of feeling imprisoned by a culture of containment was not articulated, but manifested in the patient's body. Anxiety was shown through defensive poses such as folded arms, bedsheets pulled up and held tightly around the body, tightly gripping the raised bedside rails, or nervously staring at doors and at people passing by.

These experiences reflect the reported experiences of people living with dementia more widely; the loss of freedom, restriction, anger and discomfort (Evans and Fitzgerald 2002) of being restrained (De Bellis et al. 2013). Describing the practise as 'like jail' (Powers 2001) and feeling a prisoner (Saarnio and Isola 2009). Older people within long-term community care described their resignation and acceptance of these practices (Saarnio and Isola 2009). Overall, however, there has been little exploration of the perspectives of people living with dementia on the use of these practices (Goethals et al. 2012).

Privileges and permissions

At its most subtle and everyday, beliefs about the care needs of people living with dementia, and what were believed to be appropriate care practices for them, could be seen in the forms of restraint which manifest in the most mundane aspects of their experiences of ward life. This is in contrast to the tacit permissions or 'privileges' (Stanton and Schwartz 1954; Goffman [1961] 1991; Roth 1963) afforded to other patients within these wards, which could be seen in their ability to leave the bedside without questions or sanction, in the wearing of everyday clothes, to have belongings spread out around their beds, to eat food and drink brought in from outside, to leave to buy food from the hospital mall, or to go outside and smoke a cigarette. Mundane and everyday features of hospital life, which were typically questioned and denied to people living with dementia.

Dementia as an identity was reinforced and reflected in institutional clothing, in stimuli, in day-to-day equipment and in the utensils people were permitted to have, to hold, and to use at the bedside. They became a class of patient who could quickly be identified, singled out, and returned to the bedside. This powerfully extended to include interpretations of a wide range of behaviours and actions, with almost any type of behaviour or wish, if expressed by a person living with dementia, potentially becoming viewed as problematic within the ward. Paradoxically, within these wards people living with dementia were perceived by ward staff as lacking cognitive capacity, while also wilfully disregarding the rules of these wards (as we have discussed within Chapter 6). This could mean staff verbally or physically admonished a patient for moving around on their bed, for shuffling down on their mattress, for talking across the bay, for singing, for picking up items from their tray table, or for not eating or drinking in the correct manner. The very behaviour of people with dementia was powerfully restricted, it must fit an unspoken order, with little room for personal preference or freedom of action.

As a group people living with dementia also had no choice or agency in the use of containment and restraint. Whilst ward staff would refer to 'safety' and 'risk' during this work at the bedside patients living with dementia were never involved or included in discussions about how to ensure their safety, reduce their risks of falls, or how best to be supported during their admission. Risk management and staff practices to ensure patient safety were always carried out with an expectation of compliance. Almost all behaviour exhibited by a person living with dementia could be characterised as risk, and therefore something to be contained and minimised. These organisational practices meant that people living with dementia were required to ask and to seek permission for even the most mundane and everyday activity, such as leaving the bed or bedside or walking. Frequently, such requests for permission were not regarded by staff as part of their 'appropriate tasks' (Roth and Eddy 1967: 40) or reflecting the work of the timetables, with the legitimacy of these requests always subject to adjudication.

Walking frames were required by many people living with dementia in order to walk within these wards. If they did not need them prior to their acute admission, their use was typically part of their rehabilitation following their acute admitting condition; mobility formed a key part of the discharge assessment procedures for people living with dementia. However, they were usually out of reach. Typically, there were a number of walking frames in each bay, either at the end of each bed or clustered together within one part of the bay or ward. Although some were labelled as belonging to an individual (or had been brought from home), many were shared between the patients. However, within some bays, no walking frames were present, and they had to be brought into the bays by physiotherapy and occupational therapy teams or ward staff as they felt was required during their rehabilitation and assessment work with patients at the bedside.

Because walking frames and other mobility aids were typically out of reach for patients lying in bed or sitting in their bedside chairs, this required patients to ask for the walking frame to be brought to them. In response, staff typically discouraged and always questioned requests by people living with dementia for the walking frame with '*why*' querying where they planned to go if their request was granted. Should they respond that they need to visit the toilet, staff would usually offer an alternative at the bedside, such as a bedpan or a commode. If they responded that they wanted to go home, they were likely to be told to stay in bed until 'the doctor' sees them, or similar platitudes. At the same time the patient becomes classified as a risk, either for 'falls' or for 'wandering', and leaving the ward, as in the example below:

> Alison has started to repeatedly try and get up, and the nurse keeps asking her to stay in her bed. The nurse asks Alison where she is going, Alison responds loudly that she wants to go for a horse ride. The nurse keeps insisting that Alison stay in her bed. This continues until a member of the therapy team passes the bay. She interrupts the nurse and tells her that Alison is OK to get up and walk around. She has been assessed and it is safe for her to do so, providing she uses a frame. She had been using one the previous day. After the therapist leaves, the nurse does not get a frame. Instead she helps Alison out of bed and chaperones her to the toilet, holding on to her arm to keep her upright. Once at the toilet the nurse tells Alison she will get her a 'clean nappy'. Alison requests that she brings her wash bag so can clean up, which the nurse does.
>
> After she is done in the bathroom, a frame has been brought for Alison by the therapy team. Alison walks past me and stops to introduce herself to me, shakes my hand, she was very funny and warm. She does not want to go back on the bay or to the bed; instead, she is standing in the corridor and resting on the frame, talking to those passing by enthusiastically, although her speech is

> quite incoherent. Alison is fast when she walks using the frame, but also wobbles from side to side which makes the nursing staff panic and reach out to her. The physiotherapy team are happy for her to walk with the frame, encouraging her to get used to it as she will be going home with one, but the nurses won't let her. They panic and reach out to stop her every time she moves, the risk of patient falls seems to be a massive fear for them, only the bed or chair is seen as safe. Alison is quite happy and content standing in the corridor, but the nursing staff will not let her stay there. They soon guide her back to her bedside chair, where she sits and becomes very quiet.
>
> (Site D day 4)

The inaccessibility of mobility assistance (the walking frame) was a strategy to contain patients living with dementia at the bedside and minimise risk, yet at the same time it created a new risk. Once a patient's request had been denied or delayed because it was not viewed as safe, appropriate, or a priority, the person typically continued to try to leave the bedside unaided. For example, patients living with dementia would typically use their hands to attempt to move around their bed, or would resort to using the unstable bedside tray table (which were always on wheels) to lean on to assist them, creating real risks of falling as they attempt to reach their walking frame.

Institutional cultures of restraint

Chair alarms, and sensor mats placed on the seats of bedside chairs (and occasionally attached to beds), were widely used within these wards (although not all) to monitor the movements of people living with dementia. During our observations they were only ever used to monitor people living with dementia, and were not put in place for any other patient group. These institutionally mandated interventions were categorised as 'safety measures' and associated with the policies of improving safety and preventing 'falls' in people living with dementia. These alarms were typically highly sensitive and triggered by small movements, such as someone slightly adjusting their position in their chair, producing a loud, extremely high-pitched, blaring or pulsing alarm. It was common for these alarms to become activated seemingly randomly and multiply across a bay, adding to the noise of the ward, and becoming an accepted part of the wider soundscape. If there were regular patterns of 'false' alarms, staff would quickly stop hearing these as urgent and it became a less pressing priority to respond, and occasionally stopped hearing them altogether; however, they remained highly distressing and disorienting for the person living with dementia.

Here, the alarms attached to the bedside chairs within this bay were so sensitive that they were triggered not only when the person got up from the chair, but in response to any movement, such as a person shifting their position in the chair. In response, this nurse instructs this patient living with dementia, to stop triggering the alarm attached to his chair. However, to do this he must remain perfectly still, for, as she points out, 'If you wiggle it will go off'. However, at no point does she (or the wider team) consider this request unreasonable. She expects compliance, expecting him to remain unmoving in the chair all afternoon.

It is lunchtime and the team set down the trays of lunch for everyone in the bay. One of the loud alarms attached to the chair goes off again, 'NANANANANA'… even though no one has moved or got up from their chair. The team go to the bedside of one patient and check his chair alarm, or 'movement monitor', and re-sets it. I now realise that all four people in this bay have these movement monitors attached to their chairs. None of them appeared to move at all- but even when they make a small movement or wriggle in their seat they now seem to go off, they seem far too sensitive. I now see there are pads on their seats attached to little boxes under the chair and some have an additional wire attached by a clip on their pyjama top. Another patient leans forward in the chair to start eating his lunch and the alarm goes off: 'NANANANANA'. A senior nurse in blue comes in to check on the alarm, but it has already stopped. As she is about to leave it goes off again: 'NANANANANA'. She checks the box under the chair. She then goes over to the first patient to say 'Hello' and as she does this his alarm goes off again. And the alarm on a second patient also goes off. Both alarms are now blaring out as they try to eat their lunch. 'NANANANANANANANA…'

Another nurse comes into the bay and re-sets the alarms. As she does this she explains: 'You are sitting on a pad and if you wiggle it will go off!'

It goes off again 'NANANANA…'

One patient asks 'Turn it off, nurse!'

'I will try but I can't promise anything' and this nurse re-sets the alarm and leaves.

(Site C day 4)

The patient clearly asks for this to end, 'Turn it off nurse'. For the nurse, however, this cannot happen, and she re-sets the alarm. This demonstrates the pervasive impacts of restraint. These practices could quickly transform from what may be introduced as a reasonable safety measure, into something far more restrictive for the patient. In practice, we found that their use reflects the organisational cultures, to support the expected norms and priorities of these wards, and to ensure the wider timetabled work can continue. Of note is that servicing the technology of these alarms became a key focus for this team.

The use of chair alarms demonstrates a key feature of the restraint practices we observed; they quickly became mundane, and everyday features of ward life. They are thus viewed as accepted, taken-for-granted routine aspects of the organisation and delivery of bedside care for people living with dementia.

The chair alarm goes off and the male student nurse heads over. Karen has just moved and shifted position in her bedside chair and because of the loud beeping she has taken the alarm box from the hook on the side of her chair and has it in her hands. She is now anxiously fiddling with it and shaking it and trying to make it stop. The alarm is very loud and fills the bay with noise.

He quickly strides over and stands over her and takes it from her hands. He snaps at her and seems very exasperated: 'Leave it!'

He takes it from her hands, re-sets it and hooks it back onto her chair.

(Site E day 11)

These technologies magnified the institutional concerns about the status of people living with dementia. The chair alarms triggered confusion and fear in patients, who typically did not associate the alarm with their movement. They also incited panic in staff, who in the moment, interpreted their role as managing these alarms, responding to these technologies of care rather than the patient's needs.

Hospitals have legal obligations to protect patients from harm (Human Rights Act 1998) and the care of people living with dementia in hospital is, of course, governed by complex legal regimes via *either* the Deprivation of Liberty Safeguards (DoLS) order or Section 2 and/or Section 5 the Mental Health Act 1983 (MHA). Formally, these authorise hospitals (and long-term care settings) to deprive a person of their liberty. This allows staff to act in ways they believe is in the best interests of the patient and is widely used to prevent patients living with dementia from leaving the institution on the basis that they lack capacity for decision-making in their own interests. These tools include the use of detention. Importantly, the procedural safeguards contained within DoLs (an individual's mental capacity and 'best interests' to be independently assessed, independent advocates and representatives appointed, and access to the Court of Protection) were intended to support the person in understanding their rights and ensure that any detention, restrictions, or restraint, could be reviewed and challenged.

However, within these ward cultures, we found these complex and bureaucratic legal safeguards had become transformed, through everyday practice, to inform and support the everyday cultures of restraint. The application of these legal regimes at the bedside varied widely from ward to ward. Typically, these bureaucratic mechanisms were only used when the more everyday methods of containment, restriction, and restraint had 'failed', typically because their use had prompted further resistance or agitation in the person living with dementia and the individual was now viewed as disruptive to the wider work of the ward. On some wards, however, DoLs would be put in place as a standard part of the admissions process for a person living with dementia (or for staff to assume they are already in place and acted accordingly). On other wards, they were used infrequently or not at all.

Although there is currently limited evidence to establish the full scale and extent of these practices and their impacts on people living with dementia within the acute setting (Evans et al. 2003), we do know that over half of people subject to a DoLs authorisation are people living with dementia (NHS Digital 2019). Across these wards we found wide variations in practices, and this may, to some extent, reflect their complexity and the institutional structures that support its use.

Cultures of containment in maintaining the timetables

As we have discussed in Chapter 5, the threat of 'falling behind' was powerfully felt and routinely observable within these wards and it was usual for staff to feel that their timetable was slipping. In response, staff typically prioritised approaches that would allow timetabled tasks of care at the bedside to continue without interruptions. This meant that they drew on a variety of techniques that would reduce the opportunity for other care needs that were viewed as highly variable, unpredictable or time consuming.

A key unplanned and highly variable patient need was continence care. To align this unpredictable, but essential patient need within these timetables, staff typically used a range of continence technologies that could be used to contain the person and at the bedside, and to manage and contain it within the existing timetables of bedside care.

Across all these wards it was usual practice for people living with dementia to be wearing continence pads. While these were referred to as 'pads', they were usually large wrap-around adult diapers, rather than the more discreet commercially available pads. Staff would occasionally call these a 'nappy', including in front of patients. The systematic use of continence pads for this group across these wards and sites meant that the majority of people living with dementia were encouraged to stay at the bedside to use these continence products, or to use a 'pan' or 'bottle' in bed or a commode at the bedside, behind the curtain. Walking to the bathrooms was always viewed as being both high-risk and time-consuming. Using a commode, a 'stedy' or 'rotunda' to take them to the bathroom was viewed an activity that could significantly delay and disrupt the routine timetables of care. This work of helping a person to the bathroom all typically required equipment and the involvement and coordination of a number of staff, making it an additional pressure and constraint on the ward team.

It was extremely common for people living with dementia (and other older people) to call for assistance and to specifically request support to go to the bathroom. However, staff typically interpreted these requests as neither urgent nor a legitimate need. In response, they would often ask patients to wait or to remind them that they were wearing a continence pad that they could use (which, of course, goes against the powerfully embodied knowledge that this must not happen). Such actions would be followed up with instructions to 'stay' sitting down, or to 'get back' into bed. As in the case below, the team rationalised that continence care did not need to be a priority during this shift, because '*They all have pads on so it is OK*' (site E). This meant that for the group who had been placed in continence pads, staff rarely felt it was legitimate to prioritise, allow, or support the person living with dementia to walk to the bathroom.

Here, although this person insisted on going to the bathroom, this was not seen as an appropriate request or a priority by the team. It was only when this patient was able to verbally and repeatedly express her urgency and demand support to go to the bathroom that the team responded. She becomes increasingly anxious, begs, and pleads with the team as she becomes increasingly distressed by the urgency of her need. However, extra team members were required and there was always a delay in gathering members of the team to support this, which caused huge amounts of anxiety for the person with an urgent need and for the team.

> The healthcare assistant is carrying out the observation round for Zoe. Zoe is sitting in her chair, wearing a cotton nightgown and red hospital issue socks, which means the thick bandages wrapped all around her lower legs and shins

are visible. She begs with the healthcare assistant that she needs to go to the bathroom: 'I need to go NOW please. Please...'

The healthcare assistant leans over her and says: 'I need someone to help me [she gestures to indicate that they are short staffed]. You will have to wait.'

'Please I need to wee... please, please.'

The healthcare assistant explains to me that they have only just finished the wash round for everyone and that it is almost lunchtime, but 'They all have pads on so that is OK'.

Zoe continues 'Please, ignore everyone else.' She is now very distressed.

A nurse from outside the wards hears this and offers to help her.

'I need to pee NOW!'

The team start gathering things together.

'We are coming, Zoe.'

They wheel the commode next to her and put a frame in front of her for stability. They give her clear instructions as they transfer her from her chair to the commode.

'Lift your feet, stand tall for me.'

They have not closed the screen and she has her continence pants down and it sitting on the commode in full view. Her tiny bandaged legs do not reach the floor as she sits there.

The healthcare assistant emphasises: 'You are not on the toilet so don't go yet.'

She is sitting on the commode but there is no disposable bowl underneath. They wheel her to the bathroom opposite.

(Site E day 9)

Although this person could, and was able to, ask for help, many people living with dementia did not feel able to ask, were embarrassed to ask (many whispered their needs to staff or to us at the bedside), or were unable to quickly articulate their continence needs to the team as they worked in the wider bay or ward. Access to the bathroom was a common and pressing anxiety for people living with dementia and we were often asked to relay messages of need and urgency to the teams. In the context of maintaining timetabled care schedules and reacting to the pressures of the ward, staff had to continually make decisions and judgements of need and urgency throughout their shifts, with the use of continence technologies one approach to the containment of people living with dementia and the timetables.

Containment, restriction, restraint, and cascade iatrogenesis

Of course, ensuring patients received clinical interventions and essential treatment was a key focus within the everyday work of the wards. It was extremely common for people living with dementia to pull out medical equipment attached to their bodies such as pulling out IV ports, pulling at catheter tubes and pulling off oxygen masks. Typically, staff recognised these patient responses to the equipment secured to their body as a feature of their dementia diagnosis and an action without underlying meaning or purpose, and typically tightened and further secured the equipment in place. This could also take the form of tucking in the sheets tightly so that this limited the person's movement within the bed as a way to contain them, by keeping their arms under the sheets (if someone was pulling at an IV port as in this case) or placing their hands over the sheets (if someone had been pulling at their catheter tube). However, it was rare for staff to consider or look for an underlying reason.

In the example below, Michael has repeatedly pulled out his IV drip during the night and in response the team firmly resecured it as part of his essential care and to try to make sure that he cannot detach it again. Even though he is clearly physically very weak, across two shifts he continued to try and remove it (and indeed succeeded on several occasions); however, neither teams consider that there may be an underlying reason for his tenacity, strength, and determination to remove this equipment from his body.

> 8.10 a.m. Everyone appears to be asleep. Michael is lying totally still, his head lying back on the pillows, he still has his glasses on and is staring up at the ceiling. He has a mobile drip inserted in his left arm and the team from the earlier shift reported that he had pulled out the drip from his left arm the previous night and they had to put it in again. This has happened again and there is some fluid spilt around his bed and a yellow 'Caution: Wet Floor' sign placed in the area around his bed. He is partially covered in a thin sheet with his bare feet sticking out and they look very cold. He continues to lie very still holding firmly onto the raised side bars that are on either side of his bed. He starts to fiddle with and then tried to pull the IV line out of his arm. but it looks as though it has been very firmly and securely re-attached. There is a thick layer of bandage tightly wound around it covering half of his arm. He is unable to pull it out, but he keeps trying.
>
> (Site A day 5)

There was no discussion of the potential for any underlying causes such as pain or distress, and this is attributed to his dementia. As we have discussed, however, this was also viewed by staff as a wilful rejection of essential care. So begins the cycles of escalation or 'looping', of steadily increasing restrictions of the person living with dementia with the repeated replacement of the IV held in place by the team applying further layers of bandages, which, in turn, could potentially contribute to his deteriorating condition, the cascade of decline of the person, who becomes increasingly distressed and determined to remove it. These patterns of restraint, distress, and decline, in people living with dementia were everyday and ordinary occurrences within these wards, to the extent that they were typically viewed as natural and inevitable, and viewed within these cultures as an unstoppable progression of complications and deterioration in this patient group.

Outsourcing restraint

We found that at both the organisational and the bedside levels, the restraint of people living with dementia was so common as to be a defined role, an aspect of care with its own remit that could and should be outsourced. While within these hospitals there were often small groups of highly skilled dementia specialist workers, these services were typically stretched to cover an entire hospital or Trust population. Instead they relied extensively on the use of external agency carers (or, when available, student nurses) to provide one-to-one care to people living with dementia. As discussed at the start of this chapter, such action is commonly referred to as a patient being 'specialed' and the staff member is referred to as 'specialing' a patient or bay.

In patient notes, the language around 'specialing' varies, but it often refers to 'enhanced care' or 'one to one care', which suggests the delivery of focused and therapeutic care. What we observed instead was a role that focussed on the close supervision and restriction of the person at the bedside to enable the wider ward team to continue with the organisation and delivery of timetabled care to the rest of the ward, uninterrupted by what was viewed as the additional and unpredictable needs of people living with dementia. These contemporary practices of 'specialing' more closely reflect its use historically within psychiatric care (Stanton and Schwartz 1954). Whilst this may not have been the original intention of this intervention within these contemporary wards, it has become a standard part of their organisational cultures and practice. We found that the role of the one-to-one carer was typically to simply sit close to, or even directly opposite from, the patient and to watch, contain, restrict, and restrain them, keeping the person living with dementia within their 'island', either in bed or sitting in their bedside chair in isolation from the wider ward.

Although we observed a small number of one-to-one carers who did focus on getting to know the person with which they spent a whole shift, there was typically little attempt at companionship, interaction, or bedside care, tailored to meet their care needs or evidence of its 'enhancement' to meet their specific needs. Interactions between the one-to-one carer and the patient rarely occurred outside of responding to a person's attempts to stand, walk, or 'wander'. Instead, the patient and one-to-one carer would typically sit through a shift (typically a 12-hour shift), watching one another in an awkward bored silence.

> Despite being lunchtime, it is very quiet on the bay. There are no buzzers or alarms or beeps, it's been like this all day. There is no sense of impending mania or staff rushing around; all you can hear is the quiet clink of cutlery on plates. The two healthcare assistants are still sitting with patients on bay 2, they have been there all shift. One of them is sitting opposite the patient, legs crossed, looking away, tapping away on an iPhone.
>
> (Site D day 4)

Clearly, it would be impossible to engage with a patient for an entire shift; however, we found that there was usually no attempt to do so. This one-to-one care had the potential to support people to walk safely within the ward, or who could engage in conversation, but were nonetheless expected to remain in their chair. There was no consideration that sitting in silence violates social norms, or that a person living with dementia may find this type of care intrusive or disturbing. Instead it seemed to further emphasise and underline cultures that viewed the person living with dementia as having a life with little potential, value, or personhood, with no need for stimuli or engagement. For the purposes of the ward, it was simply enough that the person is there, quiet, still, invisible, and contained.

Discussion

Despite their prominence within these wards, containment, restriction, and restraint, are under-examined and underreported features of bedside care within our hospitals. They were taken-for-granted features of these ward cultures, to some extent viewed as necessary for the smooth organisation and delivery of bedside care, one that appeared an ordinary, mundane, and unremarkable aspect of ward life. Importantly, our ethnographic findings echo that of the wider literature examining the care of people living with dementia internationally across a wide range of countries and care settings to the extent that these practices has been described as part of 'standard care' (Krüger et al. 2013) for people living with dementia.

The underpinning rationale for the use of all these forms of containment, restriction, and restraint were the commendable goals of ensuring patient safety and reducing risk, particularly preventing 'falls' during an admission. This was the pervasive and highly visible rationale within these wards, and staff appeared to be using these practices in response to the powerfully felt (and intuitionally mandated) pressures and the consequences for their wards (and for them personally) of a patient living with dementia in their care 'having a fall'. As noted by Coser, in describing the organisation of care for older patients within a general hospital ward, 'discipline must be particularly compelling in organisations devoted to warding off and fighting danger' (1962: 5). We also found that these practices of containment, restriction, and restraint were associated with extreme anxiety amongst ward staff of the ever-present risk of 'falling behind', of failing to meet the organisational demands of these wards and the requirement to complete bedside care to meet the timetables.

We know from the wider literature that the use of restraint for older people in long-term care leads to further dependence, falls, and incontinence (Hofmann and Hahn 2013), and associated with serious injury, extended admissions, and increased mortality (Evans et al. 2003). However, the impacts of these cultures and practices on individual people living with dementia were rarely considered by these organisations, or by the teams caring for them within these wards. The 'symptoms' attributed to dementia that ward staff (and the wider hospital organisation) viewed as the most problematic (this included resistance to timetabled care, and behaviour viewed as disruptive, inappropriate, or transgressive) were behaviours that typically resulted in the routine practices of containment, restriction, and restraint. Rarely, if ever, was there any consideration that these approaches could trigger further distress and lead to further deterioration and decline in the person.

8 Wandering the wards

Understandings of behaviour, permissions and privileges

Returning to the title of this book, we found that within the cultures of care in these wards, a key preoccupation focussed on the recognition and prevention of variants of one type of perceived behaviour, wandering the wards. The almost rhetorical question 'Where are you going?' would frequently be asked of the person living with dementia, a cheery admonishment used as the person was returned to the bedside to be contained, restricted, and restrained. People living with dementia often expressed very strong, and, as we have described, arguably reasonable and rational wishes and needs to leave their bedside, to walk within these (typically locked) wards, or to leave and return home. Ward staff rarely, if ever, seemed to consider that the person could be walking somewhere, instead always assuming these actions to be either purposeless '*wandering*', or an irrational desire to 'escape' or 'abscond' from the ward. Wandering and absconding were seen as inevitable features of a dementia diagnosis, which became applied to the wider population of older patients within these wards. At these bedsides, dementia became recognised in an older patient's resistance and refusal of care, and in behaviour viewed as disruptive, inappropriate, or transgressive. In the world of these wards, 'wandering' embodied all of these qualities.

For the person living with dementia, in their temporary role as patient, to be labelled as a '*wanderer*' is to be classified as someone acting without purpose (Algase et al. 2007). Implicit in the widespread use of this term is that it was always understood by ward teams to mean any person living with dementia who begins to stand, leave their bedside, and to walk from it, was viewed as doing so irrationally. At the same time, these actions could also be viewed as an individual's wilful disregard of the rules of these wards. Of course, people living with dementia within these wards were experiencing a range of cognitive decline and impaired capacity associated with their dementia diagnosis and the impacts of their admitting condition (as we have outlined within Chapter 4). However, ward staff (across all roles and specialisms) held far more generalised beliefs of the person as having reduced cognitive abilities, 'lost' their mental capacity to make decisions, to be highly physically dependant, have correspondingly low functionality and mobility, with further cognitive and physical deterioration expected during their admission. The recognition and attribution of dementia were typically tacit, often made at the bedside without the requirement of a formal diagnosis, or the recognition of the potential impact of their acute admitting condition on their present cognitive and physical functioning, the assessment or consideration of the patient's mobility or independence prior to their admission, nor informed by any rehabilitation goals. As we have seen, many people living with dementia within these wards appeared to be hallucinating, to be disoriented and 'confused', or experiencing delusions, and this could often be found at later stages of their admission to have a physical basis and associated with their acute condition, to hypoactive delirium or an infection. In addition, what was rarely, considered was that for the person living with dementia, 'wandering' often had purpose. This may have been walking to the bathroom, looking for someone or something, or simply for stimulation, to relieve boredom, in response to underlying fear or anxiety and to leave a stressful or frightening situation, or to break away from the restrictive confines of the bedside, or indeed to return home.

'Wandering' or 'wandering behaviours' are classified as a behavioural problem, a pathology, a disruptive (Algase et al. 1996), difficult (Hope and Fairburn 1990), troublesome (Hope et al. 1994), dangerous (Rowe 2008, Houston et al. 2011), and challenging (Lai and Arthur 2003) behavioural problem (Cipriani et al. 2014) associated with dementia and thus requiring intervention. Within these wards this was always recognised as requiring social control, with the work of containing, restricting, and restraining patients living with dementia from '*wandering*' or '*absconding*' being an everyday and ordinary part of ward life. This, of course, reflects the patients living with dementia who described their experience of ward life as a form of incarceration (within Chapter 7). Walking or walking unaccompanied within these wards was almost always discouraged and problematised as a form of behaviour that must be controlled and contained.

Although this was a significant focus in the care of people living with dementia, there was also contagion in the recognition and attribution of this category, with the established routine care practices believed to be appropriate for one group – people living with dementia – quickly becoming attached to a wider group of older people within these wards. Staff typically questioned all older patients who were walking, with the language inferring danger or as a form of '*escape*' from these wards. This was in contrast to the permissions afforded to other classes of patients, the small number of younger and working-age patients within these wards, who were unrestricted in their movements and whose freedoms provided a stark contrast within all of these wards.

> The healthcare assistant wakes a patient up for her observation and medication. As she does this, a younger man from the 'low-dependency' bay at the end of the ward walks past, just wearing his underpants. He is holding a wash bag in one hand and pushing his mobile drip attached to the IV port in his arm in the other, as he heads down the corridor to the bathroom at the end of the ward. At the same time, Kathleen is getting up from her bedside

> chair. Kathleen is 87 and was admitted for a fracture following a fall. She also has a diagnosis of dementia. Today, Kathleen is wearing a full-length dressing gown that is buttoned all the way up to her neck (it is the middle of summer and very hot in the ward). It is quilted in a soft purple fabric, covered with tiny sprigs of flowers like heather. As Kathleen does this, the healthcare assistant calls over to her: 'Where are you off to?' She responds that she is heading to the toilet (which is across the bay on the other side of the corridor) and the healthcare assistant is relieved: 'Oh I thought you were going to escape!' She goes over and helps her to reach her walking frame and stands behind her as she quietly murmurs 'I know, I know, I know…' closely shadowing her all the way to the bathroom and back. Afterwards, she turns to the healthcare assistants and smiles and says 'Thank you so much'. As the young man from the bay at the end of the ward walks back from the bathroom, still in just his underpants, the healthcare assistant gives me a look.
>
> (Site A day 1)

Throughout the work of these wards, we found such judgements being made continually about people living with dementia (and older people), their condition, and whether an activity or behaviour was legitimate and to be permitted. The younger man in this example walked up and down the ward, despite being dressed only in his underpants. However, the person living with dementia, Kathleen, is met with close control and surveillance over her own movements. The very behaviour of people with dementia was powerfully restricted, it had to fit into an unspoken order, with little room for personal preference or freedom of action and could manifest in the most mundane aspects of ward life. We have explored this in relation to the routine and long-standing practices of 'stripping' (Robb 1967, Roth and Eddy 1967) key markers of personal identity of people living with dementia (as we have discussed in Chapter 3) in contrast to the tacit permissions or 'privileges' (Stanton and Schwartz 1954, Goffman [1961] 1991, Roth 1963) afforded to other patients, particularly their movement and mobility, as we have seen in the previous Chapter 7. Instead, dementia as an identity was reinforced and reflected, in clothing, in stimuli, in day-to-day equipment, and the utensils people were permitted to have and to use at the bedside, and where they were permitted to be. They became a class of patient who could quickly be identified, singled out, and returned to the bedside.

This powerfully extended to include interpretations of a wide range of behaviours and actions, with almost any type of behaviour or wish, if expressed by a person living with dementia, potentially viewed as problematic within these wards. This could mean staff verbally admonished a patient for moving around on their chair (as we have seen in Chapter 7), for querying their medications (as we have seen with Harry in Chapter 6) or for not eating or drinking using the correct implement or in the correct manner (as we have seen with Julia in Chapter 5). The very behaviour of people with dementia was powerfully restricted, it must fit an unspoken order, the rules of these wards, with little recognition that this may prove difficult for people living with dementia or room for personal expression, preference or freedom of action.

A normal response to an abnormal world

Within these wards, 'behavioural' responses to care were typically located within the individual and attributed to their diagnosis of dementia. It was as if the person living with dementia was 'cut adrift' on an island within these wards, being viewed as a person defined essentially by their condition, existing in isolation, and as if unaffected by the social world in which they find themselves. Rarely, if ever, was there any consideration that many of those features staff recognised as dementia within these wards (resistance and refusal of care, and other responses to care delivery, which staff viewed as disruptive, inappropriate, or transgressive) not only manifested during a patient's admission, but could in fact be caused by the ward environment and created at the bedside. As Tony (who we met in Chapter 1), who is living with dementia, makes clear when discussing his recent hospital admission:

> Be aware that when people look as if they are resisting, they are not resisting *you*, they are resisting the situation they find themselves in and we need people to understand that.
>
> (November 2019)

What we were able to see from the privileged position as observers supports his experience, often what became viewed by the ward team as 'disruptive behaviour' were reasonable responses to the patient's reality and experiences of an admission. They constituted the powerful responses people living with dementia had to the organisation and delivery of their bedside care; people living with dementia do not easily fit the organisation and delivery of care within these hospital wards. In response, rather than an adaption and increased flexibility to support this significant patient group, we observed increased prescription and rigidity. The patterns of fragmented bedside care, the tightening of the timetables, the compulsive repetition that communicated and reinforced the rules of these wards, the routine work of containment, restriction, and restraint, were all apparent and everyday features of the care people living with dementia experienced.

There was a pervasive sense that because the organisational structures divided bedside work into tasks, the associated interactional work should also be straightforward and routine from patient to patient. Thus, approaches focussed on repeatedly prompting, and requiring, verbal confirmation of orientation, and recognition from the person that they were in a hospital, and why they were in the hospital. However, this denied and obscured (at both the organisational and ward levels) the complexity of caring for people living with dementia, which requires sensitive and nuanced interactional skills, particularly of listening. Non-verbal, or embodied, communication was not recognised as such, but understood and viewed in the context of these task-based approaches as resistant, disruptive, inappropriate, or transgressive behaviour to be managed and limited within these wards.

As we have explored (in Chapter 3), people living with dementia were often invisible within these wards and had to be extremely vocal and persistent if they were to make their needs known to ward staff, particularly if these needs fell outside of the timetable of the ward. All the people living with dementia we observed were trying to express themselves in some way. An expression of a care need, a continence need, or to express their autonomy and assert their own wishes and needs, an underlying anxiety or fear about home (where were their house keys or their wallet, concerns about a pet or family member) or wanting to go home.

Even though people living with dementia attempted to be heard and to have their immediate and often urgent care needs recognised by ward staff, this still often meant their needs were neither recognised nor prioritised. The needs of people living with dementia and the care they required typically did not, and could not, fit the expectations of the organisational structures shaping the work or conform to the 'rules' of these wards. The requests of people living with dementia were thus often assessed by staff to be routine, ordinary, and thus not urgent or important, but to the person were often extremely urgent, caused great distress, and had often been a request made repeatedly to many people passing their bedside. This could quickly intensify into the person repeatedly pleading and demanding recognition of their need, which typically resulted in the person experiencing increasing levels of distress. On the one hand, people living with dementia needed to persist to break through their invisibility, to make themselves heard, and for their requests to be recognised. However, this also put them at further risk of being recognised as demonstrating 'disruptive' behaviour, or viewed as wilfully disregarding the rules. Instead, it reinforced their precariousness, as individuals, as people, and patients, and the often-profound invisibility of their needs. This could have longer-term implications for their care; for example, they could become recognised as having more advanced forms of dementia, prolonging an admission, and could eventually mean that an individual could become classed as requiring institutionalisation.

We found powerful interactions between the ways in which care was organised and delivered at the bedside and the ways in which people living with dementia responded and reacted to care. These ward cultures and practices amplified both the behavioural responses from patients in rejecting them and the restricted care practices enrolled by staff in response to them. As Menzies Lyth points out, 'normal behaviour in a hospital setting would be likely to include a good deal of expression of distress and protest, a normal reaction to an abnormal setting' (1959: 185).

This suggests institutional 'looping', which Goffman described within the total institution as 'an agency that creates a defensive response on the part of the inmate takes this very response as the target of its next attack' (Goffman [1961] 1991: 41). We identified these dynamic interactions locally within these wards. The institutional cultures of recognition viewed any response (resistance to timetabled care, and behaviour viewed as disruptive, inappropriate, or transgressive) to the organisation of wards and the delivery of routine bedside care within them, as both a feature of a dementia diagnosis and as something requiring further management and control. However, these ward responses of increased prescription and rigidity (tightening the timetables, rigid and repetitive talk, and containment, restriction, and restraint) generated further distress in the person and in ward staff (for whom these practices created high levels of distress, anxiety, and the fear of 'falling behind'), which led, in turn, to further tightening, containment, and so on. These institutional cultures of care and their consequences supported and reinforced beliefs about both the classification of dementia and the recognition and application of this diagnosis and what constituted appropriate care for individuals.

We identified powerful patterns of contagion across these wards, which manifest in the expansion of the application of category of 'dementia', the routine care practices believed to be appropriate becoming applied to a wider group of older people within these wards, and patterns of significant stress and distress amongst everyone (patients and staff) within these wards, which could spread across cohorts of patients and within teams, and transfer between patients and staff at the bedside. This could lead to patterns of 'collective disturbances' (Stanton and Schwartz 1954, Coser 1962) where a 'mood sweeps in the general atmosphere… the majority of patients on a ward become upset at one time' (Coser 1962: 88), which has a long history as a phenomenon recognised within institutional life (Stanton and Schwartz 1954: 294).

Cultures that contain, restrict, and restrain ward staff

In the care of people living with dementia, 'this question of the culture in a hospital is absolutely crucial' (House of Lords House of Commons Joint Committee on Human Rights 2006–2007: 42). Our ethnography is a response to this, and throughout this book we have focussed our attention on these cultures and their consequences – the impacts of ward life for people living with dementia.

However, we found that these ward cultures powerfully restricted the actions of ward staff, particularly nursing and healthcare assistants. These organisational cultures were highly controlling, present in the compelling policies and practices regulating ward life and visible in the monitoring and recording practices dominating every aspect of routine bedside care. These organisational cultures narrowed and directed the remit of work within these wards to a focus on fulfilling that which must be recorded and measured. At the bedside, this manifested in the emphasis on completing the timetabled tasks of care and of 'not falling behind'. Throughout this book we have shown examples of the myriad ways in which the organisational cultures of these wards prioritised the timetabled order. This meant that ward staff could not see the immediate needs of people living with dementia, be it for pain relief, urgent continence needs, or assistance with food and drink, which instead became understood as 'a potential source of disruption, added labor, and disturbance' (Roth and Eddy 1967: 49) to the routine work of these wards.

We did see these cultures challenged. During every ward rotation it was clear that ward staff worked hard through intense 12-hour shifts to support their patients and colleagues, and witnessed the anxiety, stress, and exhaustion associated with it – also a consistent feature of ward life. Every shift there were staff who took shorter breaks or stayed to support the next team. These ward staff challenged the norms of a dominant culture, talked about 'team work' and said that 'We have to support each other', but the value of their contribution and approach quickly (as we will see in the next example) became lost and overpowered by the dominant cultures, norms, and rules of these wards.

We observed ward staff regularly try person-centred approaches, spending time with or responding more closely to the needs of their patients living with dementia. However, we also saw that these approaches would be monitored and censured by their colleagues and senior staff, and by other teams entering these wards. There was a constant surveillance of both the self and the close monitoring of colleagues that reinforced the rules of these wards. Here a healthcare assistant is caring for three men living with dementia cohorted together within a single bay. Michael, Bill, and Peter had been admitted the previous day and since then have been repeatedly trying to stand up and walk, to 'wander', and leave the bay, which the team have discouraged. In response, this healthcare assistant takes the time to sit and talk to them, and actively encourages other staff to join her. She sets up games for the men to play as a group, including a 'race night' with a simulation of horse races, played through hand-held devices and a TV screen (we had never seen it on this ward before, nor would see it again). For several hours, the staff and the patients are having fun together. However, a nurse leading the medication round and the nurse in charge of the ward both appear and reprimand the team; this is not 'proper' work. Finally, the arrival of the medical team brings this to an abrupt end. The consultant publicly admonishes the healthcare assistant for delaying his timetable and demands that the patients are returned immediately to their beds. The team learn that this is not part of the culture here and are quickly reassigned to fulfilling the timetabled tasks of the ward.

> As I begin observing the bay, Michael is standing up, and is practising walking using a frame with two young physiotherapists, while Peter is also on his feet and walking with a frame so that he can reach the bathroom. Bill keeps trying to stand as well, and is told repeatedly to sit back down by one of three healthcare assistants who rotate in and out of the bay over a ten minute period. One of the healthcare assistants is very engaged, speaking to all the men, and rearranging the bay's furniture so that the men's chairs are close to one another, in the centre of the bay rather than up against the wall. The other healthcare assistants are less engaged, supervising these patients, but not speaking to them. This new seating arrangement feels more communal than normal, and the patients seem happy with the arrangement. When Peter and Michael return to their chairs, they are practically sitting in the middle of the room. Several staff, four healthcare assistants and a nurse are talking in the entrance to the bay, frequently interrupting themselves to remind Bill and Peter to sit down. Otherwise the atmosphere is unusually convivial and friendly for this or compared to any other unit.
>
> Michael and Peter begin to talk about a pair of socks. They are on Michael's tray table, but Peter keeps on lifting them up. They both seem quite engaged and one of them asks the healthcare assistant about watching TV. The healthcare assistant says they don't have a TV, but instead of leaving them, she sits and begins a conversation about the sort of programmes they usually like to

> watch. The healthcare assistant reminds Peter that he has 'had a fall' and that is why she is sitting with him. In a friendly tone, she explains that she does not want him to fall again. She is now essentially spinning plates to keep all the patients living with dementia in this bay seated, but she is assisted now by the presence of a visitor with one of the patients and the arrival of another healthcare assistant.

The healthcare assistant's approach here stands out against the usual routines within this ward (and many others), where interactions with patients living with dementia were typically limited to instructions and to reorient them to their situation – 'YOU. ARE. IN. HOSPITAL!' – during the delivery of timetabled care. Instead this healthcare assistant and her colleague, partially helped by this being an otherwise unusually quiet and under-capacity ward, are being proactive, talking to their patients and keeping them sitting, through engaging and connecting with them. As the discussion continues, one of the healthcare assistants remembers there is a TV, and she leaves to find it.

> A monitor is wheeled onto the bay and has been placed in front of Peter and Michael. It is a modified tablet inside a wooden fascia to give it the appearance of a mid-century television, complete with knobs and dials. While they remain with Peter and Michael, the two healthcare assistants begin to busy themselves trying to figure out how the TV works, talking through the various settings. They spend ten minutes doing this, gradually excluding Michael and Peter.
>
> Eventually, the monitor comes to life, and Peter and Michael draw in closer, until the monitor prompts for a wi-fi password. None of the staff on this ward know what the password is or who to ask. At this point one of the visitors comes over, and takes a look at the monitor. The healthcare assistant tells him that they have 'had it for years', but it has never been turned on before, and nobody knows how it works.

That this monitor has never been used before is not unusual. As we have described (within Chapter 2), these types of resources were rarely used and within the majority of these wards they were neatly packed away, pristine or gathering dust, remaining in their boxes, locked away in cupboards. Such resources do not reflect ward priorities, nor are their use prescribed or organisationally quantifiable. In bringing the monitor onto this bay, the two healthcare assistants end up spending close to an hour with the three men, one of whom was previously been 'specialed' (as we have discussed in detail in Chapters 4 and 7). In spending time with these patients, Peter and Bill no longer attempt to stand up or leave, to 'wander', and the team are quickly able to resolve other issues in the moment, such as when Bill thinks he has lost his socks. This bay is now unusually calm; however, it becomes quickly apparent in the comments made within the ward that this degree of engagement is not considered to be 'proper' work or recognised as care within this ward.

> As the two healthcare assistants continue to chat with the three men, they get the monitor working, fiddling with it until it begins to play a selection of pre-recorded horse races. The picture is terrible, but the men, particularly Michael, are enthralled. As this happens, a nurse comes on to the bay to do the timetabled medication rounds. She jokes with one of the healthcare assistants, quipping 'and what did *you* do at work today!'; however, it is clear from her tone that she does not approve. The medicine round passes without incident for Peter and Michael, who are sitting staring at the monitor.
>
> Not long after this the ward sister (who is in charge of the ward) passes through the ward and sees what is happening the bay for the first time that shift. She immediately admonishes the two healthcare assistants for 'just sitting there'. She tells them that it does not take two of them to watch one patient. One of the healthcare assistants then leaves and goes to another part of the unit, but the first healthcare assistant remains, sitting on the floor between Peter and Michael. She keeps resetting the horse races for the men to watch.

While the work of the healthcare assistants in engaging with and spending time with these patients living with dementia, is not valued by the senior staff on this ward (notably all who made their disapproval known were of a higher rank in the professional hierarchy of this ward, with the higher the rank the more forcibly this disapproval was made known), it is of clear value to these men who are all living with dementia:

> The healthcare assistant flicks through the settings of the monitor to see what else there is on it. None of the dramas, such as a Basil Rathbone-style Sherlock Holmes story, keep their attention, but an animation of pigs racing and the videos of horse racing keep them entertained, especially when it is accompanied by old-fashioned fast-paced commentary. The healthcare assistant goes over asks Bill if he would like to come and watch the horse racing with them. He nods, so she pushes Michael's bed to one side and then literally drags Bill, still in his big bedside chair, across the bay, sitting him next to Peter and Michael. Bill now has a massive smile on his face. Bill really gets into it, pointing and smiling. Peter still attempts to stand occasionally, but otherwise they are all calm. A physiotherapist walks past and jokes that we all look like a little social group. When one of the nurses at the station is told about the 'pig racing' she doesn't believe it and joins them to sit with Bill and watch the monitor. She then offers him some soluble medicine as they watch together and he drinks this without any objections.

The success the healthcare assistants have in these interactions, engaging with and entertaining their patients over a couple of hours, seems to reduce the levels of anxiety, tension, and boredom, we had typically observed within this bay, and also supported the delivery of timetabled care. Two medication rounds pass with no resistance, despite all three men previously resisting all forms of bedside care and regularly attempted to leave the bedside in response to it. However, the organisational culture of this ward was unable to recognise the value in their work. It is made clear to all that this is not 'proper' care or reflect the work expected of this team, and that it does not belong within this ward:

> At half past two the medical team arrive on the unit for their timetabled bedside rounds. The consultant is clearly unimpressed with the set up on this bay. He commands the healthcare assistant to get Peter back into his bed so that they can do their rounds, stating that he will not examine them in the middle of the bay. He then turns around and apologises to the visitors on the unit, and apologises for the 'the state of the place'. Michael and Bill remain in their chairs, still watching the racing, but all of the staff leave and return to delivering timetabled tasks at the bedside.
>
> Bill immediately begins to ask for the racing again. He can't see it because the consultant has drawn the curtain around Peter's bed with the monitor behind it. When the consultant and his team leave the bay they nonchalantly move on with no thought for these men, leaving the monitor facing the wall, so that no one can see it. A new healthcare assistant takes over care on this bay. She sits between Peter and Michael but looks bored. The conversation is stilted then stops. The men begin to look very bored and restless.
>
> (Site D day 6)

These experiences and the underlying (and legitimate) fears of being reprimanded by senior staff was widespread, and contributed powerfully to the lack of conversation, interaction, and engagement with patients, and reflects long-standing institutional cultures where 'staff and patients are strictly segregated' (Rosenhan 1973: 254). Throughout out time on these wards we had few examples of staff appearing to feel able or that it was legitimate aspect of their role to spend time sitting, talking, and listening to patients. Talk spanning the boundary between staff and patients felt powerfully 'restricted' (Goffman [1961] 1991: 19). Conversation, or listening to patients, appeared to have no recognised organisational value or status within the work of these wards; and did not appear to be permitted unless formally stipulated. It was typically only something to be seen within these wards when formally prescribed, and carried out by specialist services and workers, such as Dementia Care Workers or Meaningful Activity Workers who were 'prescribed' to a patient by a member of the medical team or a senior member of the nursing team. Thus, interaction becomes the role and remit of these specialist roles and teams, not the work of these wards. Conversation or spending time with a patient, so important for people living with dementia within this fast-paced, alien and bewildering setting, was not recorded, quantified care, so lacked any validity or value.

These organisational approaches appeared to devalue work that could not be easily quantified, measured, or recorded within the present system, work that has been crudely described as 'compassionate' care and 'person-centred' care, but which was invisible to these systems of surveillance. These ideologies and commitments to 'patient-oriented' (Coser 1962: 31) care that emphasises a 'whole-patient' approach (Roth and Eddy 1967: 78) and the failure of institutions to support these approaches in the organisation and delivery of work, has a long history (Coser

1962, Roth and Eddy 1967); 'patient-centred' care has long been viewed as the desirable and dominant paradigm for the organisation and delivery of care within hospitals (Weston 2001, Kitson et al. 2013). More recently, this has developed into the goal of 'person-centred care', the requirement for caregivers to recognise the individual is at the heart of contemporary care (rather than caring for a patient or a condition), has been held as a high watermark in the provision of high-quality care for people living with dementia (Brooker 2004). Prato et al.'s (2018) study suggests that although hospital staff understand the value of focusing on the person receiving care, there is uncertainty in how to achieve this within acute wards.

The highly skilled work, the detailed interactional expertise, flexibility, and slower pace, required to provide high-quality bedside care for people living with dementia is currently not recognised, quantified, or mandated, within the task-based and fast-paced structures of care delivery, or in the metrics used to assess care quality within these wards. Yet, as we have discussed, the recognition of the centrality of highly skilled bedside care, particularly work that prioritises and values seeing the person, the monitoring and surveillance of their condition at the bedside, is vital in the prevention of a cascade of decline in the person living with dementia, that can result in further functional decline, dependency, institutionalisation, and avoidable death during an acute admission.

For people living with dementia, their care needs were often embodied and only apparent in subtle signs that could be identified in their body language and changes in behaviour that indicated an underlying need, for example, when patients looked uncomfortable, distressed, displayed potentially defensive or repetitive body language, or became silent and withdrawn. We found that these early subtle signs could usually be traced to later patterns of more entrenched distress. Caring for people living with dementia requires sensitive and nuanced interactional skills, particularly of listening and the recognition of embodied communication, which requires a slower pace. Yet these were skills that were not recognised nor valued by these institutional cultures, which emphasised pace, urgency, and the requirement to deliver care in a particular format, to a set order, and to a set time.

Importantly, for staff, recognising but not feeling able or allowed to respond to these underlying patient needs during the timetabled work of these wards was associated with emotional and physical burnout. In response, they asked for simple interventions, techniques, and training, that they could implement within their practice and their wards without having to seek 'permission' from the wider hospital administrative and executive systems. Many nurses describe to us the intractability and resistance of these wider hospital systems with their clearly demarcated hierarchies, grading of roles and chain of command, which they experienced daily, and viewed as holding back any innovations within their ward by enforcing complex and rigid processes of permissions, paperwork, and multiple systems of recording. As one nurse in charge of a ward put it, her frustration visible, during a discussion of how to improve care for older people living with dementia within her ward:

> How can we make these changes when I still can't get permission to put a nail in the wall to put a clock up in the ward! [Site A]

Cultures of change: Interventions intensify and reinforce current cultures

Within all these wards and across the organisational levels of these hospitals, we found powerful cultures that rejected change and reinforced understandings that the person (or their dementia) was viewed as at fault rather than the setting itself (see also Kitwood 1993, Borbasi et al. 2006). This supported understandings and expectations that we found to be prevalent and well-rehearsed amongst all these hospitals, that people living with dementia obstructed the smooth running of the work of these wards, as this team told us, when there is no one with dementia here 'we can get on with the tasks in hand, it's much easier' (Site C).

A key impact of these prevailing cultures was the belief that there were – or should be – other wards within these hospitals that could support the needs of people living with dementia. In response, there have been ongoing developments and expansion of the creation of wards with admission criteria established on the grading and organising of older patients. These wards have labels such as COTE (care of the elderly), RAID (rapid assessment, interface and discharge), CI (cognitive impairment) and Frailty (a category related to elderly patients perceived to have an elevated risk of injury and decline) – all categories of patients and sites of care that have emerged to replace the former older peoples and geriatric specialities.

Across these wards and institutions, we found a powerful reification of technological solutions, and their promissory potential to transform the detection, recognition, and care of 'dementia' at the bedside. All of these wards used some form of signage and symbols displayed on the semi-public admission boards and attached to the patient's bedside to indicate 'dementia'; to 'alert busy staff' that the patient they were caring for was also a person living with dementia. However, the use of these interventions without education supporting understandings of appropriate care for people living with dementia, or the adaption and increased flexibility required organisationally to support this significant patient group, these interventions appeared to further reinforce the already deeply entrenched ward cultures of care. These cultures continued to emphasise increased prescription and rigidity, patterns of fragmented bedside care, the tightening of the timetables, the compulsive repetition that communicated and reinforced the rules of the ward, and the routine work of containment, restriction, and restraint, which continued to be everyday features of the care people living with dementia experienced. In turn, these everyday experiences of precariousness experienced by patients living with dementia informed what types of patients were valued within these wards, further reinforcing their place within the organisation and priorities of these wards. We found that the use of such signage promoted significant misunderstandings of appropriate care for people living with dementia, contributing to further reinforce the invisibilities they experienced within these wards (Featherstone et al. 2019).

Ward staff are used to a steady stream of such initiatives, care bundles, and new technologies, and campaigns entering their wards; however, although these interventions were usually considered to be 'a good thing', typically they are not grounded in evidence and failed to recognise the potential ways in which they would be received, interpreted, and incorporated within these resilient ward cultures.

These 'innovations' were typically institutional policies that took the form of additional paperwork or organisational systems, and thus were unsurprisingly viewed by ward staff as adding to their workload and further overcrowding and intensifying the timetables of care. In addition, their implementation would rarely occur without a subsequent process of transformation and subversion, nor sustained in the long term within these wards. This can be observed in the rarely used day rooms, the dementia-friendly spaces, the gadgets that staff cannot operate, the rarely consulted 'This is me' forms, the misaligned signage, the computer stations gathering dust, and the storage rooms full of redundant technology and broken machinery. The priorities and the powerfully felt everyday routines and timetables of these organisational cultures quickly prevailed.

Regardless of these ongoing transformational projects, it is surprising how few fundamental changes in organisation and delivery of care have actually taken place. Despite the increasing and changing demands and expectations of their services, within these acute wards there is widespread fear and anxiety in considering change, which can lead, in turn, to further 'intensifying of current attitudes and reinforcing existing practice' (Menzies Lyth p.81).

Reversing the established patterns of decline in people living with dementia during an acute admission has typically focused on the identification, interaction, and prevention of specific adverse events and injuries and conditions associated with this decline (such as 'falls', sepsis, hospital acquired infections, and delirium) and the development of the array of new types of wards for older patients we have described. However, we need an increased focus on providing detailed and robust understandings of the role the hospital environment itself plays in generating, exacerbating, or increasing these risks, and the impacts the tightly structured task-based bedside care has in informing these poor outcomes, which is currently poorly understood.

The powerful impacts of routine care delivered at the bedside, by the large number of nurses, healthcare assistants, medical teams, allied health professionals, and auxiliary staff working within these wards, which require complex and highly skilled interactional work, have typically been downplayed and have remained relatively invisible within these debates, awareness campaigns, and transformational projects. Yet there is evidence to suggest that for people living with dementia, the characteristic cascade of decline they experience during a hospital admission may be closely associated with care at the bedside, particularly the work of seeing the person, and the routine monitoring and surveillance at the bedside (Thornlow et al. 2009). Our analysis helps to confirm this important finding and supports the clinical significance of our detailed ethnographic work.

Continuities of the ward and involvement of people living with dementia

During this ethnography we have involved carers and people living with dementia at every stage of our research, consulting them throughout. This consultation led us in developing our approaches, identifying appropriate methods, our strategies of access, consent and ethics committee approvals, our emergent analysis, the potential for interventions and priority setting for future projects. We have done this through their involvement in our research grants as co-applicants, and as members of our steering committees, but also by hosting meetings, workshops, festivals, and events where we have shared our research, recognising that it is important for us to listen. People living with dementia and carers must have a voice in directing our research. They tell us that we have helped in some small way to provide 'a tremendous sense of self-worth' and 'healing from invisibility'. We believe we are the ones who have gained, in knowledge, in awareness, understanding, and through collaboration and lasting friendships. We are answerable to a funding body, but ultimately we are working for the people living with dementia and the carers who have been with us and supported us – we are ultimately answerable to them to make visible their experiences, and to understand why these cultures of care continue, so that we can inform improvements in everyday care.

They have been our guides, and our mentors, and have allowed us into their worlds. Throughout our work, we have borne witness to their experiences and have tried to be faithful to their experiences and to make them visible, throughout this book.

As we have described, we found remarkable continuity with the hospital ethnographies of the 1950s, 1960s and 1970s (Stanton and Schwartz 1954, Caudill 1958, Lyth 1959, Coser 1962, Roth 1963, Roth and Eddy 1967, Zerubavel 1979). We also found remarkable stability and resilience in the organisation and delivery of care across these wards, despite the apparent widespread changes in ward demographics, technologies, awareness, and competencies. Although our ethnography and all we present within this book is necessarily incomplete and partial, witnessing and recording their consequences for people living with dementia and over many months, we know too well the precariousness of identity and the quickly made assessments and judgements of social worth within the institution, which suggests we should all take note. Dementia is indiscriminate, and none of us can be certain we will remain unaffected.

References

Albert, M.S., De Kosky, S.T., Dickson, D., Dubois, B., Feldman, H.H., Fox, N.C., & Phelps, C.H. (2011) 'The diagnosis of mild cognitive impairment due to Alzheimer's disease: recommendations from the National Institute on Aging-Alzheimer's Association workgroups on diagnostic guidelines for Alzheimer's disease', *Alzheimer's & Dementia*, 7 (3): 270–279.

Algase, D.L., Beck, C., Kolanowski, A., Whall, A., Berent, S., Richards, K., & Beattie, E. (1996) 'Need-driven dementia-compromised behavior: an alternative view of disruptive behavior', *American Journal of Alzheimer's Disease*, 11 (6): 10–19.

Algase, D.L., Moore, D.H., Vandeweerd, C., & Gavin-Dreschnack, D.J. (2007) 'Mapping the maze of terms and definitions in dementia-related wandering', *Aging & Mental Health*, 11 (6): 686–698.

Alzheimer's Society. (2009) *Counting the Cost: Caring for People with Dementia on Hospital Wards*. London: Alzheimer's Society.

Alzheimer's Society. (2016) *Fix Dementia Care: Hospitals*. London: Alzheimer's Society.

American Psychiatric Association. (2013) *Diagnostic and Statistical Manual of Mental Disorders*, Fifth Edition (DSM-5). Arlington: American Psychiatric Association.

Ang, S.Y., Bakar Aloweni, F.A., Perera, K., Wee, S.L., Manickam, A., Lee, J.H.M., Haridas, D., Shamsudin, H.F., & Chan, J.K. (2015) 'Physical restraints among the elderly in the acute care setting: prevalence, complications and its association with patients' characteristics', *Proceedings of Singapore Healthcare*, 24 (3): 137–143.

Archibald, C. (2006) 'Meeting the nutritional needs of patients with dementia in hospital', *Nursing Standard*, 20 (45): 41–45.

Bagot, M. (2018) 'Hospital bed block shock – social care chaos sparks new surge in elderly patients stuck on wards', *The Mirror*, 18 September, p. 1.

Bandak, A. & Janeja, M.K. (2018) 'Introduction: worth the wait', in M.K. Janeja & A. Bandak (eds), *Ethnographies of Waiting: Doubt, Hope and Uncertainty*. London: Bloomsbury, pp. 1–39.

Banicek, J. (2010) 'How to ensure acute pain in older people is appropriately assessed and managed', *Nursing Times*, 106 (29): 14–17.

Boenink, M. (2016) 'Biomarkers for Alzheimer's disease: searching for the missing link between biology and clinic', in M. Boenink, H. van Lente, & E. Moors (eds), *Emerging Technologies for Diagnosing Alzheimer's Disease*. Health, Technology and Society. London: Palgrave Macmillan.

Borbasi, S., Jones, J., Lockwood, C., & Emden, C. (2006) 'Health professionals' perspectives of providing care to people with dementia in the acute setting: toward better practice', *Geriatric Nursing*, 27 (5): 300–308.

Bowker, G.C. & Star, S.L. (2000) *Sorting Things Out: Classification and Its Consequences*. Cambridge: MIT Press.

Bradley, L. & Rees, C. (2003) 'Reducing nutritional risk in hospital: the red tray', *Nursing Standard*, 17 (26): 33–37.

Bredthauer, D., Becker, C., Eicher, B., Koczy, P., & Nikolaus, T. (2005) 'Factors relating to the use of physical restraints in psychogeriatric care: a paradigm for elder abuse', *Zeitschrift fur Gerontologie und Geriatrie*, 38: 10–18.

Brindle, N. & Holmes, J. (2005) 'Capacity and coercion: dilemmas in the discharge of older people with dementia from general hospital settings', *Age & Ageing*, 34 (1): 16–20.

Brooker, D. (2004) 'What is person-centred care in dementia?, *Reviews in Clinical Gerontology*, 13 (3): 215–222.

Bunn, F., Goodman, C., & Burn, A.M. (2015) 'Multimorbidity and frailty in people with dementia', *Nursing Standard*, 30 (1): 45–50.

Buse, C. & Twigg, J. (2014) 'Looking "out of place" analysing the spatial and symbolic meanings of dementia care settings through dress', *International Journal of Ageing and Later Life*, 9 (1): 69–95.

Buse, C.E. & Twigg, J. (2015) 'Clothing, embodied identity and dementia: maintaining the self through dress', *Age, Culture, Humanities*, 40 (2): 340–352.

Butler, J. (1997) *Excitable Speech: A Politics of the Performative*. London: Routledge.

Capezuti, E., Strumpf, N.E., Evans, L.K., Grisso, J.A., & Maislin, G. (1998) 'The relationship between physical restraint removal and falls and injuries among nursing home residents', *The Journals of Gerontology Series A: Biological Sciences and Medical Sciences*, 53 (1): M47–M52.

Capezuti, E., Strumpf, N., Evans, L., & Maislin, G. (1999) 'Outcomes of night time physical restraint removal for severely impaired nursing home residents', *American Journal of Alzheimer's Disease*, 14 (3): 157–164.

Care Quality Commission. (2011) *Dignity and Nutrition Inspection Programme: National Overview*. London: The Stationery office

Care Quality Commission. (2014) *The State of Health Care and Adult Social Care in England in 2013/14*. London: The Stationery Office.

Caudill, W.A. (1958) *The Psychiatric Hospital as a Small Society*. Cambridge: Harvard University Press.

Charmaz, K. (2014) *Constructing Grounded Theory*. London: Sage.

Charmaz, K., & Mitchell, R. G. (2001) Grounded theory in ethnography. *Handbook of ethnography*, 160–174.

Chuang, Y.H. & Huang, H.T. (2007) 'Nurses' feelings and thoughts about using physical restraints on hospitalized older patients', *Journal of Clinical Nursing*, 16 (3): 486–494.

Cipriani, G., Lucetti, C., Nuti, A., & Danti, S. (2014) 'Wandering and dementia', *Psychogeriatrics*, 14 (2): 135–142.

Cohen, L. (1998) *No Aging in India: Alzheimer's, the Bad Family, and Other Modern Things*. Berkeley, CA: University of California Press.

Cohen-Mansfield, J. & Mintzer, J.E. (2005) 'Time for change: the role of nonpharmacological interventions in treating behavior problems in nursing home residents with dementia', *Alzheimer Disease & Associated Disorders*, 19 (1): 37–40.

Coleman, E.A. (1993) 'Physical restraint use in nursing home patients with dementia', *Journal of the American Medical Association*, 270 (17): 2114–2115.

Collins, N., Blanchard, M.R., Tookman, A., & Sampson, E.L. (2010) 'Detection of delirium in the acute hospital', *Age and Ageing*, 39 (1): 131–135.

Corbin, J. & Strauss, A. (1990) 'Grounded theory research: procedures, canons and evaluative criteria', *Zeitschrift Fur Soziologie*, 19: 418–427.

Coser, R.L. (1962) *Life in the Ward*. East Lansing, MI: Michigan State University Press.

Cramer, H., Hughes, J., Johnson, R., Evans, M., Deaton, C., Timmis, A., Hemingway, H., Feder, G., & Featherstone, K. (2018) '"Who does this patient belong to?" Boundary work and the re/making of (NSTEMI) heart attack patients', *Sociology of Health & Illness*, 40 (8): 1404–1429.

Creditor, M.C. (1993) 'Hazards of hospitalization of the elderly', *Annals of Internal Medicine*, 118 (3): 219–223.

Daykin, N. & Clarke, B. (2000) '"They'll still get the bodily care". Discourses of care and relationships between nurses and health care assistants in the NHS', *Sociology of Health & Illness*, 22 (3): 349–363.

De Bellis, A., Mosel, K., Curren, D., Prendergast, J., Harrington, A., & Muir-Cochrane, E. (2013) 'Education on physical restraint reduction in dementia care: a review of the literature', *Dementia*, 12 (1): 93–110.

Department of Health. (2009) *Living Well with Dementia: A National Dementia Strategy*. London: Department of Health.

Desantis, J., Engberg, S., & Rogers, J. (1997) 'Geropsychiatric restraint use', *Journal of the American Geriatrics Society*, 45 (12): 1515–1518.

Dewing, J. (2007) 'Participatory research: a method for process consent with persons who have dementia', *Dementia*, 6 (1): 11–25.

Digby, R., Lee, S., & Williams, A. (2017) 'The experience of people with dementia and nurses in hospital: an integrative review', *Journal of Clinical Nursing*, 26 (9–10): 1152–1171.

Drennan, D. (1992) *Transforming Company Culture*. London: McGraw-Hill Book Company.

Evans, D. & Fitzgerald, M. (2002) 'Reasons for physically restraining patients and residents: a systematic review and content analysis', *International Journal of Nursing Studies*, 39 (7): 735–743.

Evans, L.K. & Strumpf, N.E. (1989) 'Tying down the elderly', *Journal of the American Geriatrics Society*, 37 (1): 65–74.

Evans, D., Wood, J., & Lambert, L. (2003) 'Patient injury and physical restraint devices: a systematic review', *Journal of Advanced Nursing*, 41 (3): 274–282.

Featherstone, K. & Atkinson, P. (2012) *Creating Conditions: The Making and Remaking of a Genetic Condition*. Oxford: Routledge.

Featherstone, K., Atkinson, P., Bharadwaj, A., & Clarke, A.J. (2006) *Risky Relations: Family and Kinship in the Era of New Genetics*. Oxford: Berg.

Featherstone, K., Latimer, J., Atkinson, P., Pilz, D., & Clarke, A.J. (2005) 'Dysmorphology and the spectacle of the clinic', *Sociology of Health and Illness*, 27 (5): 551–574.

Featherstone, K., Northcott, A., & Bridges, J. (2019) 'Routines of resistance: an ethnography of the care of people living with dementia in acute hospital wards and its consequences', *International Journal of Nursing Studies*, 96: 53–60.

Fleck, L. (1979) *Genesis and Development of a Scientific Fact*. Chicago: University of Chicago Press.

Foucault, M. ([1975] 1995) *Discipline & Punish: The Birth of the Prison*. New York: Vintage.

Fox, R.C. (1959) *Experiment Perilous: Physicians and Patients Facing the Unknown, Glencoe*. New Brunswick, IL: Free Press.

Francis, R. (2013) *Report of the Mid Staffordshire NHS Foundation Trust public inquiry*. London: The Stationery Office.

George, J., Long, S., & Vincent, C. (2013) 'How can we keep patients with dementia safe in our acute hospitals? A review of challenges and solutions', *Journal of the Royal Society of Medicine*, 106 (9): 355–361.

Gerace, A., Mosel, K., Oster, C., & Muir-Cochrane, E. (2013) 'Restraint use in acute and extended mental health services for older persons', *International Journal of Mental Health Nursing*, 22: 545–557.

Gibbons, K. (2016) 'NHS crisis deepens as bed blocking costs NHS £6bn – delays push hospitals to breaking point', *The Times*, 12 August, p. 1.

Gladman, J., Porock, D., Griffiths, A., Clissett, P., Harwood, R.H., Knight, A., Jurgens, F., Jones, R., Schneider, J., & Kearney, F. (2011) 'Better mental health: care for older people with cognitive impairment in general hospitals'. Final report. National Institutes for Health Research Service Delivery and Organisation Programme.

Glaser, B. & Strauss, A. (1967) *The Discovery of Grounded Theory*. London: Weidenfeld & Nicolson.

Goethals, S., Dierckx de Casterlé, B., & Gastmans, C. (2012) 'Nurses' decision-making in cases of physical restraint: a synthesis of qualitative evidence', *Journal of Advanced Nursing*, 68 (6): 1198–1210.

Goffman, E. ([1961] 1991) *Asylums: Essays on the Social Situation of Mental Patients and Other Inmates*. London: Penguin Books.

Goffman, E. ([1963] 2009) *Stigma: Notes on the Management of Spoiled Identity*. New York: Simon and Schuster.

Goldberg, S.E., Whittamore, K.H., Harwood, R.H., Bradshaw, L., Gladman, J.R.F., & Jones, R. (2012) 'The prevalence of mental health problems amongst older adults admitted as an emergency to a general hospital', *Age & Ageing*, 41 (1): 80–86.

Green, J. (1998) 'Commentary: grounded theory and the constant comparative method', *BMJ*, 316 (7137): 1064.

Griffiths, P. (2013) 'A necessary evil? Nurses and the use of physical restraints in the care of older people' *International Journal of Nursing Studies.*

Gupta, S. & Warner, J. (2008) 'Alcohol-related dementia: a 21st-century silent epidemic?', *The British Journal of Psychiatry*, 193 (5): 351–353.

Hacking, I. (2007, April) Kinds of people: Moving targets. In *Proceedings - British Academy* (Vol. 151, p. 285). Oxford: Oxford University Press.

Hillman, A. & Latimer, J. (2017) 'Cultural representations of dementia', *PLoS Medicine*, 14 (3): e1002274.

Hofmann, H. & Hahn, S. (2013) 'Characteristics of nursing home residents and physical restraint: a systematic literature review', *Health, Risk and Society*, 9 (4): 3012–3024.

Holmes, J. (1999) 'The detection of psychiatric factors predicting poor outcome in elderly hip fracture patients'. MD thesis, University of Leeds.

Hope, R.A. & Fairburn, C.G. (1990) 'The nature of wandering in dementia: a community-based study', *International Journal of Geriatric Psychiatry*, 5 (4): 239–245.

Hope, T., Tilling, K.M., Gedling, K., Keene, J.M., Cooper, S.D., & Fairburn, C.G. (1994) 'The structure of wandering in dementia', *International Journal of Geriatric Psychiatry*, 9 (2): 149–155.

Houghton, C., Murphy, K., Brooker, D., & Casey, D. (2016) 'Healthcare staffs' experiences and perceptions of caring for people with dementia in the acute setting: qualitative evidence synthesis', *International Journal of Nursing Studies*, 61: 104–116.

House of Lords/House of Commons Joint Committee on Human Rights. (2007) *Report of 18th session 2006/7 The Human Rights of Older People in Healthcare*. London: The Stationary Office

Houston, A.M., Brown, L.M., Rowe, M.A., & Barnett, S.D. (2011) 'The informal caregivers' perception of wandering', *American Journal of Alzheimer's Disease & Other Dementias*, 26 (8): 616–622.
Hughes, R. (2008) 'Toward restraint-free care for people with dementia', *British Journal of Neuroscience Nursing*, 5 (5): 222–226.
Hynninen, N., Saarnio, R., & Isola, A. (2015) 'Treatment of older people with dementia in surgical wards from the viewpoints of the patients and close relatives', *Journal of Clinical Nursing*, 24 (23–24): 3691–3699.
Jervis, L.L. (2001) 'The pollution of incontinence and the dirty work of caregiving in a US nursing home', *Medical Anthropology Quarterly*, 15 (1): 84–99.
Jones, J., Borbasi, S., Nankivell, A. and Lockwood, C. (2006) 'Dementia related aggression in the acute sector: is a Code Black really the answer?', *Contemporary Nurse*, 21 (1): 103–115.
Kirk, H. (1992) 'Geriatric medicine and the categorisation of old age; the historical linkage', *Ageing & Society*, 12 (4): 483–497.
Kirkevold, Ø. & Engedal, K. (2004) 'A study into the use of restraint in nursing homes in Norway,' *British journal of nursing*, 13 (15): 902–905.
Kitson, A., Marshall, A., Bassett, K., & Zeitz, K. (2013) What are the core elements of patient-centred care? A narrative review and synthesis of the literature from health policy, medicine and nursing. *Journal of Advanced Nursing*, 69 (1): 4–15.
Kitwood, T. (1993) 'Towards a theory of dementia care: the inter-personal process', *Ageing and Society*, 13: 51–67.
Koch, T. & Iliffe, S. (2010) 'Rapid appraisal of barriers to the diagnosis and management of patients with dementia in primary care: a systematic review', *BMC Family Practice*, 11 (1): 52.
Koch, S., Nay, R., & Wilson, J. (2006) 'Restraint removal: tension between protective custody and human rights', *International Journal of Older Peoples Nursing*, 1: 151–158.
Kontos, P.C. (2004) 'Ethnographic reflections on selfhood, embodiment and Alzheimer's disease', *Ageing & Society*, 24 (6): 829–849.
Kontos, P.C. (2005) 'Embodied selfhood in Alzheimer's disease: rethinking person-centred care', *Dementia*, 4 (4): 553–570.
Kontos, P.C. (2012) 'Rethinking sociability in long-term care: an embodied dimension of selfhood' *Dementia*, 11 (3): 329–346.
Kontos, P. & Martin, W. (2013) 'Embodiment and dementia: exploring critical narratives of selfhood, surveillance, and dementia care', *Dementia*, 12 (3): 288–302.
Kontos, P.C. & Naglie, G. (2007) 'Bridging theory and practice: imagination, the body, and person-centred dementia care', *Dementia*, 6 (4): 549–569.
Krüger, C., Mayer, H., Haastert, B., & Meyer, G. (2013) 'Use of physical restraints in acute hospitals in Germany: a multi-centre cross-sectional study', *International Journal of Nursing Studies*, 50 (12): 1599–1606.
Lai, C.K.Y. & Arthur, D.G. (2003) 'Wandering behaviour in people with dementia', *Journal of Advanced Nursing*, 44 (2): 173–182.
Lane, C. & Harrington, A. (2011) 'The factors that influence nurses' use of physical restraint: a thematic literature review', *International Journal of Nursing Practice*, 17 (2): 195–204.
Launer, L.J. (2011) 'Counting dementia: there is no one "best" way', *Alzheimer's & Dementia*, 7 (1): 10–14.
LeCouteur, D.G., Doust, J., Creasey, H., & Brayne, C. (2013) 'Political drive to screen for pre-dementia: not evidence based and ignores the harms of diagnosis', *British Medical Journal*, 347 (9): f5125.

Lee, D.T.F., Chan, Tam, E.P.Y., & Yeung, W.S.K. (1999) 'Use of physical restraints on elderly patients: an exploratory study of the perceptions of nurses in Hong Kong', *Journal of Advanced Nursing*, 29 (1): 153–159.

Lejman, E., Westerbotn, M., Pöder, U., & Wadensten, B. (2013) 'The ethics of coercive treatment of people with dementia', *Nursing Ethics*, 20 (3): 248–262.

Liukkonen, A. & Laitinen, P. (1994) 'Reasons for uses of physical restraint and alternatives to them in geriatric nursing: a questionnaire study among nursing staff', *Journal of Advanced Nursing*, 19 (6): 1082–1087.

Lloyd, J., Schneider, J., Scales, K., Bailey, S., & Jones, R. (2011) 'Ingroup identity as an obstacle to effective multiprofessional and interprofessional teamwork: findings from an ethnographic study of healthcare assistants in dementia care', *Journal of Interprofessional Care*, 25 (5): 345–351.

Lock, M. (2013) *The Alzheimer Conundrum: Entanglements of Dementia and Aging*. Princeton, NJ: Princeton University Press.

Long, D., Hunter, C., & Van der Geest, S. (2008) 'When the field is a ward or a clinic: hospital ethnography', *Anthropology & Medicine*, 15 (2): 71–78.

Macaulay, S. (2018) 'The broken lens of BPSD: why we need to rethink the way we label the behavior of people who live with Alzheimer disease', *Journal of the American Medical Directors Association*, 19 (2): 177–180.

Manthorpe, J. & Iliffe, S. (2016) 'The dialectics of dementia'. Social Care Workforce Research Unit, King's College London, London.

Manthorpe, J., Samsi, K., Campbell, S., Abley, C., Keady, J., Bond, J., Watts, S., Robinson, L., Warner, J., & Iliffe, S. (2013) 'From forgetfulness to dementia: clinical and commissioning implications of diagnostic experiences', *British Journal of General Practice*, 63 (606): e69–e75.

Marini, G., Vulcano, V., & Costantini, S. (1998) 'Dementia and restraint', *Archives of Gerontology and Geriatrics*, 26: 301–304.

Menzies Lyth, I. ([1959] 1988) *Containing Anxiety in Institutions: Selected Essays*. London: Free Association Books.

Merrick, J. (2015) 'Bed Blockers cost the NHS £287 million', *The Independent*, 23 March, p. 1.

Meyer, G., Köpke, S., Haastert, B., & Mühlhauser, I. (2009) 'Restraint use among nursing home residents: cross-sectional study and prospective cohort study', *Journal of Clinical Nursing*, 18 (7): 981–990.

Minnick, A.F., Mion, L.C., Johnson, M.E., Catrambone, C., & Leipzig, R. (2006) 'Prevalence and variation of physical restraint use in acute care settings in the US', *Journal of Nursing Scholarship*, 39 (1): 30–37.

Mion, L.C., Frengley, J.D., Jakovcic, C.A., & Marino, J.A. (1989) 'A further exploration of the use of physical restraints in hospitalized patients', *Journal of the American Geriatrics Society*, 37 (10): 949–956.

Moreira, T., May, C., & Bond, J. (2009) 'Regulatory objectivity in action: mild cognitive impairment and the collective production of uncertainty', *Social Studies of Science*, 39 (5): 665–690.

Morrison, R.S. & Siu, A.L. (2000) 'A comparison of pain and its treatment in advanced dementia and cognitively intact patients with hip fracture', *Journal of Pain and Symptom Management*, 19 (4): 240–248.

Moyle, W., Borbasi, S., Wallis, M., Olorenshaw, R., & Gracia, N. (2010) 'Acute care management of older people with dementia: a qualitative perspective', *Journal of Clinical Nursing*, 20 (3–4): 420–428.

Moyle, W., Olorenshaw, R., Wallis, M., & Borbasi, S. (2008) 'Best practice for the management of older people with dementia in the acute care setting: a review of the literature', *International Journal of Older People Nursing*, 3 (2): 121–130.
Mukadam, N. & Sampson, E.L. (2011) 'A systematic review of the prevalence, associations and outcomes of dementia in older general hospital inpatients', *International Psychogeriatrics*, 23 (3): 344–355.
Muñiz, R., Gómez, S., Curto, D., Hernández, R., Marco, B., García, P., Tomás, J.F., & Olazarán, J. (2016) 'Reducing physical restraints in nursing homes: a report from Maria Wolff and Sanitas', *Journal of the American Medical Directors Association*, 17 (7): 633–639.
Nakanishi, M., Okumura, Y., & Ogawa, A. (2018) 'Physical restraint to patients with dementia in acute physical care settings: effect of the financial incentive to acute care hospitals', *International Psychogeriatrics*, 30 (7): 991–1000.
Natan, M.B., Akrish, O., Zaltkina, B., & Noy, R.H. (2010) 'Physically restraining elder residents of long-term care facilities from a nurses' perspective', *International Journal of Nursing Practice*, 16 (5): 499–507.
National Audit Office. (2007) *Improving Services and Support for People Living with Dementia*. London: The Stationery Office.
NHS Digital. (2019) '*New figures on Deprivation of Liberty Safeguards released*', https://digital.nhs.uk/news-and-events/news/new-figures-on-deprivation-of-liberty-safeguards-released (accessed 5 March 2020).
Norman, R. (2006) 'Observations of the experiences of people with dementia on general hospital wards', *Journal of Research in Nursing*, 11 (5): 453–465.
O'Connor, D., Horgan, L., Cheung, A., Fisher, D., George, K., & Stafrace, S. (2004) 'An audit of physical restraint and seclusion in five psychogeriatric admission wards in Victoria, Australia', *International Journal of Geriatric Psychiatry*, 19 (8): 797–799.
O'Grady, S. (2018) 'Scandalous waste of health cash – Bed blocking costs NHS £3 billion a year', *The Daily Express*, 16 June, p. 1.
Office of National Statistics. (2019) Death registration summary tables', https://www.ons.gov.uk/peoplepopulationandcommunity/birthsdeathsandmarriages/deaths/bulletins/deathsregistrationsummarytables/2018 (accessed 5 March 2020).
Petersen, R.C., Doody, R., Kurz, A., Mohs, R.C., Morris, J.C., Rabins, P.V., Ritchie, K., Rossor, M., Thal, L., & Winblad, B. (2001) 'Current concepts in mild cognitive impairment', *Archives of Neurology*, 58 (12): 1985–1992.
Pinkert, C. & Holle, B. (2012) 'Menschen mit Demenz im Akutkrankenhaus', *Zeitschrift Für Gerontologie Und Geriatrie*, 45 (8): 728–734.
Poole, M., Bond, J., & Hughes, J.C. (2014) 'Going home? An ethnographic study of assessment of capacity and best interests in people with dementia being discharged from hospital', *BMC Geriatrics*, 14 (1): 56.
Powers, B.A. (2001) 'Ethnographic analysis of everyday ethics in the care of nursing home residents with dementia: a taxonomy', *Nursing Research*, 50 (6): 332–339.
Prato, L., Lindley, L., Boyles, M., Robinson, L., & Abley, C. (2019) 'Empowerment, environment and person-centred care: a qualitative study exploring the hospital experience for adults with cognitive impairment', *Dementia*, 18 (7–8): 2710–2730.
Robb, B. (1967) *Sans Everything: A Case to Answer*. London: Nelson.
Rosenhan, D.L. (1973) 'On being sane in insane places', *Science*, 179 (4070): 250–258.
Rosenhan, D.L. (1975) 'The contextual nature of psychiatric diagnosis', *Journal of Abnormal Psychology*, 84 (5): 462–474.
Rosenhan, D.L. (1979) When does a diagnosis become a clinical judgment?. In *Clinical Judgment: A Critical Appraisal* (pp. 45–56). Dordrecht: Springer.

Roth, J. (1963) *Timetables: Structuring the Passage of Time in Hospital Treatment and Other Careers*. Indianapolis, IN: Bobbs Merrill.

Roth, J. & Eddy, E.M. (1967) *Rehabilitation for the Unwanted*. New York: Atherton Press.

Rothschild, J.M., Bates, D.W., & Leape, L.L. (2000) 'Preventable medical injuries in older patients', *Archives of Internal Medicine*, 160 (18): 2717–2728.

Rothschild, J.M., Hurley, A.C., Landrigan, C.P., Cronin, J.W., Martell-Waldrop, K., Foskett, C., Burdick, E., Czeisler, C.A., & Bates, D.W. (2006) 'Recovery from medical errors: the critical care nursing safety net', *The Joint Commission Journal on Quality and Patient Safety*, 32 (2): 63–72.

Rowe, M. (2008) 'Wandering in hospitalized older adults: identifying risk is the first step in this approach to preventing wandering in patients with dementia', *AJN, The American Journal of Nursing*, 108 (10): 62–70.

Russ, C.T., Shenkin, S.D., Reynish, E., Ryan, T., Anderson, D., & MacLullich, A.M.J. (2012) 'Dementia in acute hospital inpatients: the role of the geriatrician', *Age and Ageing*, 41 (3): 282–284.

Saarnio, R. & Isola, A. (2009) 'Use of physical restraint in institutional elderly care in Finland: perspectives of patients and their family members', *Research in Gerontological Nursing*, 2 (4): 276–286.

Sampson, E.L., Blanchard, M.R., Jones, L., Tookman, A., & King, M. (2009) 'Dementia in the acute hospital: prospective cohort study of prevalence and mortality', *The British Journal of Psychiatry*, 195 (1): 61–66.

Sampson, E.L., Gould, V., Lee, D., & Blanchard, M.R. (2006) 'Differences in care received by patients with and without dementia who died during acute hospital admission: a retrospective case note study', *Age and Ageing*, 35 (2), 187–189.

Sampson, E.L., Leurent, B., Blanchard, M.R., Jones, L., & King, M. (2013) 'Survival of people with dementia after unplanned acute hospital admission: a prospective cohort study', *International Journal of Geriatric Psychiatry*, 28 (10): 1015–1022.

Sampson, E.L., White, N., Lord, K., Leurent, B., Vickerstaff, V., Scott, S., & Jones, L. (2015) 'Pain, agitation, and behavioural problems in people with dementia admitted to general hospital wards: a longitudinal cohort study', *Pain*, 156 (4): 675–683.

Saukko, P. (2008) *The anorexic self: A personal, political analysis of a diagnostic discourse*. New York: SUNY Press.

Scheltens, P. & Rockwood, K. (2011) 'How golden is the gold standard of neuropathology in dementia?' *Alzheimer's & Dementia*, 7 (4): 486–489.

Simpson, R., Slutskaya, N., & Hughes, J. (2012) 'Gendering and embodying dirty work: men managing taint in the context of nursing care', in R. Simpson, N. Slutskaya, P. Lewis, & H. Höpfl (eds), *Dirty Work*. London: Palgrave Macmillan, pp. 165–181.

Stanton, A.H. & Schwartz, M.S. (1954) *The Mental Hospital: A Study of Institutional Participation in Psychiatric Illness and Treatment*. New York: Basic Books.

Star, S.L. (1999) 'The ethnography of infrastructure', *American Behavioral Scientist*, 43 (3): 377–391.

Suddaby, R. (2006) 'From the editors: What grounded theory is not', *Academy of Management Journal*, 49 (4): 633–642.

Suzman, R.M., Willis, D.P., & Manton, K.G. (1996) *The Oldest Old*. Oxford: Oxford University Press.

Swaffer, K. (2014) 'Dementia and prescribed disengagement', *Dementia*, 14 (1): 3–6.

Tadd, W., Hillman, A., Calnan, M., Bayer, T., & Read, S. (2011) 'Right place – wrong person: dignity in the acute care of older people', *Quality in Ageing and Older Adults*, 12: 33–43.

Thornlow, D.K., Anderson, R., & Oddone, E. (2009) 'Cascade iatrogenesis: factors leading to the development of adverse events in hospitalized older adults', *International Journal of Nursing Studies*, 46 (11): 1528–1535.

Tolson, D., Smith, M., & Knight, P. (1999) 'An investigation of the components of best nursing practice in the care of acutely ill hospitalized older patients with coincidental dementia: a multi-method design', *Journal of Advanced Nursing*, 30: 1127–1136.

Twigg, J. (2000) 'Carework as a form of bodywork', *Ageing and Society*, 20 (4): 389–412.

Twigg, J. (2010) 'Clothing and dementia: a neglected dimension?', *Journal of Ageing Studies*, 24 (4): 223–230.

Twigg, J. & Buse, C.E. (2013) 'Dress, dementia and the embodiment of identity', *Dementia*, 12 (3): 326–336.

United Kingdom: Human Rights Act 1998 [United Kingdom of Great Britain and Northern Ireland], 9 November 1998.

van der Geest, S. & Finkler, K. (2004) 'Hospital ethnography: introduction', *Social Science & Medicine*, 59 (10): 1995–2001.

Voss, S., Black, S., Brandling, J., Buswell, M., Cheston, R., Cullum, S., Kirby, K., Purdy, S., Solway, C., Taylor, H., & Benger, J. (2017) 'Home or hospital for people with dementia and one or more other multimorbidities: what is the potential to reduce avoidable emergency admissions? The HOMEWARD Project Protocol', *BMJ Open*, 7 (4): e016651.

Wang, W.-W. & Moyle, W. (2005) 'Physical restraint use on people with dementia: a review of the literature', *The Australian Journal of Advanced Nursing*, 22 (4): 46–52.

Watkin, L., Blanchard, M.R., Tookman, A., & Sampson, E.L. (2012) 'Prospective cohort study of adverse events in older people admitted to the acute general hospital: risk factors and the impact of dementia', *International Journal of Geriatric Psychiatry*, 27 (1): 76–82.

Weston, W.W. (2001) 'Informed and shared decision-making: the crux of patient-centred care', *CMAJ*, 165 (4): 438–439.

Wise, J. (2010) Number of 'oldest old' has doubled in the past 25 years. *BMJ*.

Wolkowitz, C. (2006) *Bodies at Work*. London: Sage.

Wolverson, E., Birtles, H., Moniz-Cook, E., James, I., Brooker, D., & Duffy, F. (2019) 'Naming and framing the behavioural and psychological symptoms of dementia (BPSD) paradigm: professional stakeholder perspectives', *OBM Geriatrics*, 3 (4): 1–19.

World Health Organization. (1992) *The ICD-10 Classification of Mental and Behavioural Disorders*. Geneva: World Health Organization.

Xyrichis, A., Hext, G., & Clark, L.L. (2018) 'Beyond restraint: raising awareness of restrictive practices in acute care settings', *International Journal of Nursing Studies*, 86: A1–A2.

Zerubavel, E. (1979) *Patterns of Time in Hospital Life: A Sociological Perspective*. Chicago, IL: University of Chicago Press.

Zerubavel, E. (1996) 'Lumping and splitting: notes on social classification', *Sociological Forum*, 11 (3): 421–433.

Zerubavel, E. (2015) *Hidden in Plain Sight: The Social Structure of Irrelevance*. Oxford: Oxford University Press.

Zerubavel, E. (2018) *Taken for Granted: The Remarkable Power of the Unremarkable*. Princeton, NJ: Princeton University Press.

Zhavoronkov, A. & Bhullar, B. (2015) Classifying aging as a disease in the context of ICD-11. *Frontiers in Genetics*, 6: 326.

Index

For Product Safety Concerns and Information please contact our EU representative GPSR@taylorandfrancis.com
Taylor & Francis Verlag GmbH, Kaufingerstraße 24, 80331 München, Germany

www.ingramcontent.com/pod-product-compliance
Ingram Content Group UK Ltd.
Pitfield, Milton Keynes, MK11 3LW, UK
UKHW020205200926
475702UK00004B/615
* 9 7 8 1 3 5 0 0 7 8 4 5 1 *